Endomorph Diet

The Complete Guide To Drop Excess Fat, Gain Muscle, and Stay Healthy With 14 Day Meal Plan and Specific Exercises & Training Programs For Your Body Type

Tiffany Nicholas

TERMS & CONDITIONS

All Rights Reserved

No part of this cookbook may be reproduced or transmitted in any form whatsoever, electronics mechanical, including photocopying, or by any informational storage or retrieval system without expressed written, dated and signal permission from the author.

Copyright © by Tiffany Nicholas (2020)

Disclaimer

The information in this book should not be used for diagnosing or treating any health problem. Not all diet and exercise plans suit everyone. You should always consult a trained medical professional before starting a diet, taking any form of medication, or embarking on any fitness or weight-training program. The author and publisher disclaim any liability arising directly or indirectly from the use of this book.

Always follow safety and commonsense cooking protocol while using kitchen utensils, operating ovens and stoves, and handling uncooked food. If children are assisting in the preparation of any recipe, they should always be supervised by an adult. Readers are encouraged to seek professional help when is required.

This guide is for informational purposes only and the author does not accept any responsibilities for any liabilities resulting from the use of this information. While every attempt has been made to verify the information provided here, the author cannot assume any responsibility for errors, inaccuracies or omission.

TABLE OF CONTENTS

INTRODUCTION	1
ENDOMORPH BODY	5
ENDOMORPH BODY DIET	10
Endomorph Acceptable Food Items	11
Endomorph Unacceptable Food Items	12
Advantages of the Endomorph Diet	12
Disadvantages of the Endomorph Diet	13
BEST FAT BURNERS FOR ENDOMORPHS	15
CALCULATING MACRONUTRIENTS OF THE ENDOMORPH DIET	22
14 DAY SAMPLE DIET PLAN FOR ENDOMORPH BODY	28
RECIPES FOR ENDOMORPH BODY TYPE	33
Breakfast Recipes	33
Lunch recipes	66
Dinner Recipes	97
Snacks	**135**

ENDOMORPH EXERCISES — **136**
   Types of training — 136
   Endomorph Workout — 137
   7 days sample of endomorph workout plan — 151

MAINTAINING THE REQUIRED WEIGHT — **155**

CONCLUSION — **161**

INTRODUCTION

It's a hell of lots of work to lose weight and burn the gathered fat as a person with an endomorph body type. An endomorph body type is the kind of body that is easy to store fat and very difficult to lose the gathered fat. The main challenge of people with endomorph body type is the inability to shed excess body fat that was gained easily.

Some people who have endomorph body type love lifting weight to build muscle, but what they got after several weightlifting sessions is a bulky body. This is a body condition where layers of fat cover the muscles and never show the muscles in their entirety.

However, average endomorphs want to be cut and don't really want to look like the opposite of its body type-ectomorph. This body type consumes more foods than others but finds it difficult to add weight as they have higher metabolisms. Whatever muscles the ectomorph has gotten will be quickly used as body fuel, in addition to the fat stored.

Now between the endomorphs and ectomorphs is another body type known as a mesomorph. The mesomorph has perfect metabolism. The body functions are balanced between catabolism and anabolism. This set of people can easily be recognized at the gym. They don't bust their heads on the stair machine or the treadmill. They tend to do well on any weight loss diet as they can gain weight with any diet and be able to shed the calories when not needed again.

The endomorphs and ectomorphs have tried many recommended supplements and diets to get bloated, acne, a leaky gut, and many other side effects. But this book is written to solve the basic problems associated with the endomorphs. It is written to expose you to what your body entails, how to recognize your body type, the foods to eat and not to eat, and the kinds of workouts (both low and high intensity).

Not only is this book about the diet, but it also exposes you to how to calculate your macros. Why is this necessary? Once you decide the calories needed per day, you should know the amounts of calories you need per meal.

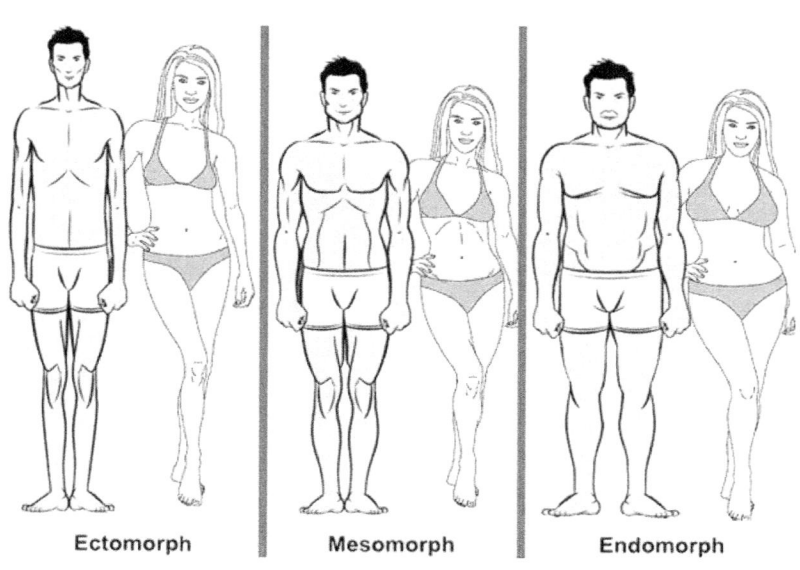

Chapter 1

ENDOMORPH BODY

Losing weight as it is added can be a daunting task for people with endomorph body type. Endomorph body is known to gain weight and keep it easy, but losing or maintaining it becomes extremely difficult due to possession of slow metabolism. Endomorphs possess less muscle mass but a higher ratio of body fat, thereby making their bodies look rounder, heavier, and curvier but are not necessarily obese.

Endomorphs tend to consume more calories compared with other body types- ectomorph and mesomorph. So they are always advised to watch their food consumption to prevent eating more calories than is necessary to burn in the body. So if you have an endomorph body and want to add 5 pounds to your weight, all you have to do is walk across to a donut shop and grab some to do the magic.

Not that people with endomorph body will not be able to maintain their health goals, but they can achieve anything they desired in as much they follow a specific diet and exercise plan explained in this book. It is not a misformed to be born with an endomorph body, as it is as a result of what we inherited from our parents. This inheritance from our parents determines whether the body will be heavier, learner, or wide hips.

The followings are the basic features of the endomorph body:

High tendency to store fat.

Thick rib cage.

Shorter limbs.

Wider waistline.

Wider hips.

Bone structure bigger.

Slow metabolism.

Apart from the endomorph body type, the other two types from the three main somatotype body types- Ectomorph and Mesomorph are explained below.

Ectomorph body consumes more foods than others, but they find it difficult to add weight as they have higher metabolisms. It is discovered that their skeleton frames are thin. Other features include;

• Bone Structure smaller.
• Narrow hips.
• Smaller joints.
• Long and lean limb.
• Long muscle bellies.
• Fast metabolism.
• Loses fat easily.

Mesomorph body is the body with more muscle and is characterized by being an hourglass-shaped body. This set of people are in between the endomorph and ectomorph as they have a lower ratio of body fat and bigger skeletal frame. Mesomorphs, unlike endomorphs, have the ability to lose weight and gain muscle easily. Feature of Mesomorphs are;

• Wide hips.
• Narrow waistline.
• Thinner joints.

- Long bellies.
- Bone Structure medium.
- Round bellies.
- Fast metabolism.
- Loses fat easily.

So the best advice to adhere to if you discovered that you have an endomorph body type is to keep a very close look at the calories you will be consuming from now on. The advice is to have a protein consumption of up to 35% per day, a 40% ratio of fat per day, and a lower amount of 25% of carbohydrates per day. With the aim of having 1,300 to 1,500 calories per day. In a nutshell, your goal is to maximize carbs and calories and have your focus on consuming lots of fiber-rich veggies.

Endomorph Hybrid Body types

Another body type that should be explained is endomorph bodies; these are types of bodies that come from the addition of DNA and bad habits over a long time. They are also known as meso-endomorphs as they are known to have larger bodies that are very strong but with no definite muscles. The best advice if you are the type is to have a combination of cardio and strength exercises, with a diet plan that will target fat loss.

Chapter 2

ENDOMORPH BODY DIET

The endomorphs are known to have more fat, and there is a strong tendency for them to have insulin resistance, so it is recommended that they consume a balanced diet with low carbohydrates to help them lose the fat. There is a professional recommendation that if the endomorph can reduce the number of carbs in the meals, it will improve insulin functions in the body within a day, and that's a great way of reducing the risk of prediabetes.

As written earlier, the best diet for endomorphs is a meal with higher amounts of fat, higher amounts of protein, and a lower amount of carbohydrates, such as the Paleo diet plan. The Paleo diet aims at fruits, meats, veggies, fish, oils, seeds, and nuts. History made us understand that our ancestors ate this Paleo

Diet when they were wandering the planet earth millions of years ago.

The Paleo diet helps the body lose fat and, at the same time, keep the energy level up.

ENDOMORPH ACCEPTABLE FOOD ITEMS

The followings are some of the acceptable food items for the endomorph diet:

Meat & Fish: Cod, Salmon, Turkey, and Chicken.

Diary: Milk and Yogurt

Fruits & Veggies: Tomatoes, Apples, Asparagus, Zucchini, Berries, spinach, Pears, romaine, Onions, and Kale.

Nuts & Seeds: Pumpkin seeds, Almonds, Sunflower seeds, Pistachios, Nut and seed butter.

Starchy vegetables & Grains: Oats, Quinoa, Sweet potatoes, Beans, Brown rice, and Squash.

ENDOMORPH UNACCEPTABLE FOOD ITEMS

The general recommendation is for the endomorphs to focus their meals on non-starchy vegetables, nonfat dairy, lean meat, and they should avoid fatty food items and refined carbohydrates.

The following food items are to be avoided:

Refined carbohydrates: White, rice, refined muffins, refined cakes, refined bread, sugars, Sweetened cereals, sweetened yogurt, and snack foods.

Fatty foods: fried foods, whole- milk, limit red meat, butter, and skinned poultry.

ADVANTAGES OF THE ENDOMORPH DIET

Not only will the endomorph diet in this book helps in losing fat, but it will also help in the improvement of health in profound ways. Ways such as lowering the risk of type 2 diabetes, heart disease, and stroke.

Following the endomorph diet plan in this book will help in adopting healthy eating habits, and the exercises added with the diet will help improve insulin activity and the loss of fat, especially visceral fat.

DISADVANTAGES OF THE ENDOMORPH DIET

Even though the endomorph diet comes with some great benefits, it also has disadvantages that prove to be challenges for some people.

The first hurdle lies in the fact that due to the body type's nature, managing the carb is very challenging as it produces excess insulin. So the hurdle is how to reduce consumption of carb, increase the healthy fats (mono-saturated fatty acids), and a good percentage of proteins.

It is very easy to tell someone or decide not to eat some set of foods due to the body's nature. But the ability to hold the decision and stop eating what's not good for the body, maintaining the best eating and lifestyle is not easy. But what should at the back of your mind is the goal set and must be reached.

Chapter 3

BEST FAT BURNERS FOR ENDOMORPHS

To the endomorphs, some supplements and ingredients are for this body type. The followings are some of the best fat-burners for endomorph body type:

Black Pepper Extract:

Black pepper extract will help the body in the absorption and uses of nutrients. There is an extract in the black pepper known as piperine. No wonder piperine is part of almost all the fitness supplements made for fat burners. It is used to increase the absorption of nutrients easily (bioavailability). The research discovered that if bioavailability is increased to 3 0000%, piperine in the black pepper will turn the fat-burning stack to a fat burner. So, if you are an endomorph, piperine is essential to help in the metabolism.

Bioperine® is one of the supplements that contained piperine, and the ratio is 95% piperine. This supplement is found to be effective and work well.

Cayenne Pepper Extract:

Cayenne pepper has a hot and spicy taste that makes it an effective way of burning fat. The extract in the cayenne pepper that takes care of the fat-burning process is known as Capsaicin. Capsaicin is a stimulant-free compound that is great for endomorphs as it helps in the burning of fats in three ways.

1. This extract has the ability to suppress appetite. This attribute will help in avoiding having extra calories during the day.

2. If Cayenne pepper extract Capsaicin is taken, it will help make you full during the meal. So the deal is to take Capsaicin before your meal, and it will help indirectly in burning fat more.

3. Another great benefit of Capsaicin is that it enhances the metabolic rate.

Capsimax® is a great brand as a supplement when it comes to Capsaicin an extract from cayenne pepper. This brand is standardized to 2% capsaicinoids.

Garcinia Cambogia:

Garcinia Cambogia originated from Asia and is featured with an outer shell that makes the source of the fat-burning advantage. There is an extract that is found inside the thick rind of Garcinia Cambogia known as hydroxycitric acid (HCA). Apart from the fact that Garcinia Cambogia is a fat burner, it's also a free stimulant. It can be taken during the day, and you should not worry if it will affect your sleep.

This acid is a special compound that will helps the endomorphs on stubborn metabolisms in three ways.

1. It helps in suppressing appetite.

2. It helps in preventing the storage of fat.

3. Hydroxycitric acid will aid an increase in the metabolic rate of the body.

Coelus Forskohlii:

Coleus forskohlii is from Thailand and Nepal. It is a powerful fat-burner that has been in existence since time immemorial. There is an extract in the Coleus forskohlii known as forskohlii. This extract greatly supports the burning of fat of endomorphs.

Forskohlii helps increase the production of a compound called cyclic adenosine monophosphate (cAMP) in the body. This compound will ensure that when the cAMP is high, the body will switch into the stored fat and use it as a fuel source. This process is just to make sure that the fatter the body uses, the leaner it becomes. Like Capsaicin, forskohlii will help the body naturally in boosting metabolism to burn more fat.

Forslean® is an excellent brand for the endomorphs, as it has an ideal dosage at 20% forskohlii. This supplement is potent, effective, and proven to work.

Green Coffee Extract:

Like green tea, green coffee beans also have a unique extract known as chlorogenic acid (CGA). The one fortunate thing about this extract is that most of its potency is lost when the beans are roasted. So your coffee cup will not have the right amount of CGA needed while drinking it.

The chlorogenic acid enhances the loss of fat in the endomorphs by forcing it to make use of the stored fat as fuel. Another work of chlorogenic acid is to increase the usage of fatty acids for the metallic processes needed every day.

To enjoy the extract, it must contain 20% CGA or more.

Green tea Extract:

Do you know that green tea is not for drinking only but also an excellent way for the endomorphs to burning their fats? Green tea has an antioxidant called epigallocatechin gallate (EGCG). This green tea extract will increase the body's rate of calorie burning and increase metabolic rate.

The professionals recommend that any supplement taken from green tea should have nothing less than 70% EGCG. It is these amounts that will trigger the right fat burning in the body. Green tea is low in caffeine but can also come in the decaffeinated form if you don't want anything to affect your sleep. If you are having nausea when taken green tea extract on an empty stomach, it is advised to check your tolerance before continuing, especially when on a fasting day.

Caffeine Anhydrous:

Caffeine is what makes you go for a cup of coffee in the morning. We all know that caffeine is a brain-booster, but some don't know that it is also a fat burner (thermogenic). One of the benefits of caffeine is that it helps in suppressing appetite while at the same time, increase the body's chances of burning calories. It can also help in preventing the body from storing fat.

One of the best forms of caffeine is Di-Caffeine. Add a molecule of malic acid to caffeine, and you will be able to increase your body's ability to digest, absorb, and digest the caffeine. Remember that the two hundred milligrams per serving are recommended per serving of caffeine in burning fat for the endomorphs.

Chromium Picolinate:

Are you looking for what will improve your digestion? Chromium is critical for the body when it comes to digestion. We all know the process- we eat. It breaks down into a usable form known as glucose. But when there is more than enough glucose in the body due to poor digestion, it will be stored in fat. But chromium Picolinate can help the body in using up the excess glucose.

So Chromium Picolinate is an excellent supplement for weight loss as it will help support the absorption and utilization of the fat burners. It is a free stimulant fat burner, and you don't have to worry about its effect on your sleep. The best Chromium Picolinate should be 1,000 mg (1 gram).

Chapter 4

CALCULATING MACRONUTRIENTS OF THE ENDOMORPH DIET

You want to lose weight, want to be more energized, or gain more muscle?

This chapter will expose you to all about macros and some free applications to calculate the needed macros if you don't want to do it manually.

Before we begin the journey, be aware that eating a healthy diet that suits your conditions and body type is more than just counting calories. It is highly recommended that you have a balanced diet that contains a variety of nutrients that will nourish your body, the energy needed, and the ability to enhance the digestive system. One of the best ways to know what and how you are eating to lose or gain weight is to track the macronutrients. Counting your calories will help you in achieving your fitness goals faster than targeting calories alone.

What are macronutrients?

Macronutrients are molecules that the human body needed in large amounts to survive. However, micronutrients are also molecules needed to survive but in small amounts like electrolytes, vitamins, and minerals.

The macronutrients are fats, carbohydrates, and proteins. Don't be disturbed by all the fads about fat. All three components are needed to survive. It is very dangerous to your health if any of the components is missing as you will be putting yourself at risk of nutrient deficiencies.

Fats

A diet that contains fat is essential for the body, as it has many responsibilities for the body. It is the function of fat to digest fat-soluble vitamins that include Vitamins A, D, E, and K, to cover the body against cold weather and to be able to withstand a long period of starvation. Not only are the above reason why fat is critical, but it also helps in protecting organs, supporting the growth of cells, and in the induction of hormone production.

Carbohydrates

The main function of carbohydrates is to provide quick energy. When we consume carbohydrates, the body will convert it to glucose (sugar) and will either be used as sugar immediately or be stored as glycogen to be used later. There is another set of carbohydrates known as complex carbohydrates, including whole grains and starchy vegetables. These sets of carbohydrates enhance the digestive system as they are very high in dietary fiber.

Protein

It is the primary function of proteins to aids the repair injuries, growth, building muscle, prevention of infections, and many more. Proteins come from amino acids that are building blocks of many structures in the body. The human body requires 20 different amino acids; nine out of the number are essential amino acids. These nine amino acids can't be produced by the body on its own but can only be gotten from food. Foods that contain the high protein are yogurt, poultry, fish, dairy products, beef, soy, and cheese. Some plant-based diet includes vegetables, starches, and beans that are also sources of proteins.

Amount of calories in each macronutrient

Fats contain 9 calories for every gram.

Carbohydrates contain 4 calories for every gram.

Proteins contain 4 calories for every gram.

What to eat as an endomorph.

The followings are the recommended ratios:

Fat: 40%

Carbohydrates: 25%

Proteins: 35%

Your aim is to have 1,300 to 1,500 calories per day.

Note: The reason for these rations is explained in chapter 1.

How to calculate macros manually?

You know what macros and how many calories they

have. The next is to know how to calculate it. The reason is that the intake ratio is in percentage, while the nutritional information is given in grams.

Assuming your daily calories is 1,500 calories per day.

And your ideal ratio is:

Fat: 40%

Carbohydrates: 25%

Proteins: 35%

Next is to times the total calories per day by the percentages.

And finally, divide the calorie amounts with calorie per gram number.

Let's do the math!

Fat: 1,500 x 0.4 = 600 (Your fats intake per day must be within this number)

Carbohydrates: 1,500 x 0.25= 375 (Your carbs intake per day must be within this number)

Proteins: 1,500 x 0.35 = 525 (Your proteins intake per day must be within this number)

So in calculating the actual gram amounts follow these steps:

Fat (9 calories per gram): 600 divides by 9 = 66.66 grams of fat

Carbohydrates (4 calories per gram): 375 divides by 4 = 93.75 gram of carbs

Protein (9 calories per gram): 525 divides by 4 = 132.25 grams of protein

But if you don't want to calculate manually, there are macronutrients calculators you can get online that will do the math for you.

1. IIFYM (https://www.iifym.com/iifym-calculator/): If It Fits Your Macros, the full name is the most comprehensive calculator for macros.

2. Katy Hearn Fit (https://www.katyhearnfit.com/macro-calculator): This calculator allows customizing your plan and choosing the number of grams of fat and protein you will like to use for your diet.

Chapter 5

14 DAY SAMPLE DIET PLAN FOR ENDOMORPH BODY

Day 1

Breakfast: Creamy-cheese Omelet

Snack: Sunflower seeds and sliced avocado

Lunch: Roasted Shrimp with cauliflower

Dinner: Spiced Chicken & Avocado Salad

Day 2

Breakfast: Sweet Potatoes Skillet

Snack: Carrots dipped in Almond butter

Lunch: Exotic Chicken Curry

Dinner: Baked Meaty Zucchini with Pesto Sauce

Day 3

Breakfast: Bacon-Egg Roll-Ups

Snack: Sliced veggies cubed cantaloupe

Lunch: Lime Avocado Salad

Dinner: Seasoned Cod Tacos & Cabbage Slaw

Day 4

Breakfast: Baked Cauliflower Hash Egg Cups

Snack: Pistachios and hummus

Lunch: Garnished Ground beef & zucchini

Dinner: Paleo Pie Dinner

Day 5

Breakfast: Cream Pancakes with Raspberries

Snack: Carrots dipped in Sunflower butter

Lunch: Curry Chicken

Dinner: Creamy Zucchini

Day 6

Breakfast: Milky Smoked Salmon Omelet

Snack: Protein shake

Lunch: Blue Cheese Salad and Steak

Dinner: Keto Tomato Soup & Chicken

Day 7

Breakfast: Cream Mushroom Breakfast Casserole

Snack: Hard-boiled egg and veggies

Lunch: Spiced Beefless Ground Beef & Riced Cauliflower

Dinner: Creamy Avocado with Bacon Omelet

Day 8

Breakfast: Baked Bacon Avocado

Snack: Salmon wrapped with lettuce

Lunch: Paleo Chicken Salad

Dinner: Creamy Chicken & Mushroom Sauce

Day 9

Breakfast: Butter Ham with Wrapped Cheddar Burrito

Snack: Hard-boiled egg Sliced Avocado

Lunch: Spicy-Sour Chicken

Dinner: Creamy Crispy Zucchini fries

Day 10

Breakfast: Milky Veggie Quiche

Snack: Sliced apple with Sunflower butter

Lunch: Creamy Keto Salad

Dinner: Spiced Beet pasta With Spaghetti

Day 11

Breakfast: Keto Herbal

Snack: Hummus and a piece of fruit

Lunch: Beef Burger & keto Sauce

Dinner: Creamy Italian Turkey Salad

Day 12

Breakfast: Seasoned Brussels Hash

Snack: Protein bar

Lunch: Milky Creamy Cauliflower

Dinner: Spaghetti Squash Shrimp

Day 13

Breakfast: Avocado with Breakfast Sausage

Snack: Carrots dipped in Sunflower butter

Lunch: Spiced Chicken & Avocado Asparagus Salad

Dinner: Spiced Avocado

Day 14

Breakfast: Frozen Veggie Acai

Snack: Sour Cream with sliced almonds

Lunch: Finger-licking Chicken salad

Dinner: Spicy Roasted Chicken

Chapter 6

RECIPES FOR ENDOMORPH BODY TYPE

BREAKFAST RECIPES

Breakfast 1

CREAMY-CHEESE OMELET

Cook Time: 15 minutes

Servings: 2

Ingredients:

4 Tablespoons Heavy Cream (whipped)

2 Big Sized Eggs

2 Tablespoons Coconut oil

3/4 Cup Cheese (mature, shredded)

Salt

Black Pepper (ground)

Topping

4 Mushrooms (sliced)

4 Cherry Tomatoes (sliced)

2 oz. baby Spinach

2 oz. Turkey

2 Teaspoons Oregano (Dried)

Preparation:

1. Combine eggs and whipped cream in a medium bowl.

2. Whisk the combination until well blended.

3. Add salt and pepper to give taste and adjust if necessary.

4. Place a non-sticking frying pan on medium heat.

5. Pour coconut oil into the frying pan to get hot.

6. Spread the shredded cheese evenly on the heated pan.

7. Make sure the cheese covers the bottom of the frying pan.

8. Fry the cheese until there are bubbles.

9. Spread the egg carefully on the cheese in the frying pan.
10. Lower the heat.
11. Don't cook the mixture for some minutes.
12. Use a spatula to divide the mixture into four portions.
13. Fill the two portions with tomatoes, mushrooms, turkey, oregano, cream cheese, and baby spinach.
14. Cook for 2 to 3 minutes more.
15. Use a spoon to lift the two portions with no other ingredient to top the twos with ingredients.
16. It will look like a hemisphere.
17. Remove them from the heat and enjoy it.

Amount per serving:

Calories 593

Total Fat 47g ; Saturated Fat 30.2g; Cholesterol 332mg; Sodium 484mg; Total Carbohydrate 14.2g; Dietary Fiber 4.6g; Total Sugars; Protein 30.8g; Vitamin D 150mcg; Calcium 422mg; Iron 7mg; Potassium 1030mg.

Breakfast 2

SWEET POTATOES SKILLET

Servings: 3

Ingredients:

1/4 kg Breakfast Sausage

2 Eggs (large)

1 Sweet Potatoes (medium)

1 Avocado (diced)

Hot Sauce

Cilantro

Raw Cheese (handful)

Preparation:

1. Preheat your oven to 400°F.

2. Transfer skillet to medium heat.

3. Pour the sausage and brown.

4. Use a slotted spoon to pick the brown sausage and allow the sweet potatoes to cook.

5. Toss the sweet potatoes into the sausage grease and allow it to get cooked and well crispy.

6. Make three holes in the pan.

7. Break gently each egg in the hole.
8. Place the skillet in the oven.
9. Bake the mixture for 5 to 8 minutes and allow the eggs to be firmed and not hardened.
10. Remove it from the oven.
11. Place avocado, cilantro, and hot sauce on top.
12. Serve and enjoy.

Amount per serving:

Calories 516

Total Fat 40.4g; Saturated Fat 11.7g; Cholesterol 181mg; Sodium 784mg; Total Carbohydrate 15.1g; Dietary Fiber 5.8g; Total Sugars 3.5g; Protein 24.1g; Vitamin D 10mcg; Calcium 88mg; Iron 2mg; Potassium 738mg.

Breakfast 3

BACON-EGG ROLL-UPS

Time: 30 Minutes

Servings: 6

Ingredients:

3 Tablespoons Milk

8 Eggs (large)

1/2 Teaspoon garlic (powder)

3 Tablespoons Milk

1 1/2 Tablespoons Butter

1 1/2 Tablespoons Chives (chopped)

18 Slices of Bacon

2 1/2 Cups Cheddar Cheese (shredded)

Preparation:

1. Combine Milk, Eggs, and garlic powder in a large bowl.
2. Mix until well combined.
3. Add salt and pepper for taste.
4. Place a non-stick skillet on medium heat and pour butter in it.

5. Heat until the butter melt.

6. Add egg mixture and scramble the mixture for some minutes.

7. Then add chives and allow it to be hot. Set aside.

8. Place six slices of bacon on a cutting board.

9. Use a spoon to pour some scrambled egg onto the cheddar cheese.

10. Then roll it tightly.

11. Do the same for other cheddar cheese and eggs.

12. Place the skillet back to the heat.

13. Put the roll-ups cheddar side of the bacon.

14. Cook and flip them over from one side to another until they turn crispy on all sides.

15. Take the skillet from the heat and remove the rolls into the plate, and enjoy

Amount per serving:

Calories 629

Total Fat 48.7g; Saturated Fat 21.8g; Cholesterol 341mg; Sodium 1733mg; Total Carbohydrate 4.4g; Dietary Fiber 0g; Total Sugars 3.2g; Protein 41.9g; Vitamin D 49mcg; Calcium 436mg; Iron 2mg; Potassium 516mg.

Breakfast 4

BAKED CAULIFLOWER HASH EGG CUPS

Time: 30 Minutes

Servings: 6

Ingredients:

1/2 Head Cauliflower (medium, cut into florets, steamed)

7 Eggs (Large)

1 Cup Cheddar (shredded)

Garlic Powder (pinch)

Pinch of Salt

2 Slices Bacon

For Serving:

Black Pepper (ground)

Chives (ground)

Preparation:

1. Preheat your oven to 375°F.

2. Pour butter or oil to grease your six muffin tin cups and place them aside.

3. Pour the steamed cauliflower into a blender and blend until it becomes a fine grain.

4. Remove the cauliflower from the blender and pour it into paper towels to get rid of the excess water.

5. Twist the paper towels until all the water is removed, and the cauliflower is dried.

6. Mix the dry cauliflower, garlic powder, cheddar, one egg, and salt well in a large bowl.

7. Pour the mixture evenly into the muffin cups.

8. Use your fingers to press the content in the tins until it becomes nests in shape.

9. Place them in the oven and bake until the edges turn to golden or 10 minutes.

10. Remove them from the oven.

11. Add bacon to the bottom of the tins.

12. Crack one egg on top of the bacon added and be sure that the yolk does not scatter.

13. Transfer the tins back to the oven and bake until the egg becomes firm or 10 to 12 minutes.

14. Remove the tins from the oven and sprinkle chives and pepper on top.

15. Serve and enjoy.

Amount per serving:

Calories 147

Total Fat 9.1g; Saturated Fat 3.3g; Cholesterol 202mg; Sodium 367mg; Total Carbohydrate 2.4g; Dietary Fiber 0.6g; Total Sugars 1.1g; Protein 13.9g; Vitamin D 18mcg; Calcium 112mg; Iron 1mg; Potassium 190mg.

Breakfast 5

CREAM PANCAKES WITH RASPBERRIES

Time: 50 Minutes

Servings: 8

Ingredients:

For Pancakes:

8 Eggs (large)

14 oz. Cottage Cheese

4 oz. Coconut oil

2 Tablespoons of Psyllium husk powder (ground)

For Topping:

2 Cups Heavy Cream (whipped)

4 oz. Raspberries

Preparation:

1. Mix cheese, psyllium powder, and eggs in a medium bowl thoroughly.

2. Allow resting for 15 minutes to become thick a little.

3. Pour the coconut oil into a non-stick skillet and place over medium heat.

4. With the aid of a large spoon, pour the egg mixture into the skillet.

5. Fry each for 3 minutes.

For Topping:

6. Pour the heavy cream into a separate bowl and whip it until it turns soft.

7. Serve the pancakes with the cream and raspberries.

8. Enjoy.

Amount per serving:

Calories 341

Total Fat 30.7g; Saturated Fat 21.1g; Cholesterol 209mg; Sodium 275mg; Total Carbohydrate 4.7g; Dietary Fiber 0.9g; Total Sugars 1.2g; Protein 13.2g; Vitamin D 31mcg; Calcium 81mg; Iron 1mg; Potassium 150mg.

Breakfast 6

MILKY SMOKED SALMON OMELET

Time: 20 Minutes

Servings: 2

Ingredients:

2 oz. Salmon (smoked)

4 Eggs (large)

2 Teaspoons Milk (low-fat)

1 Tablespoon Extra Virgin Olive oil

2 Tablespoons Fresh Basil (chopped)

1/2 Avocado (large, sliced)

Pinch of Salt

Preparation:

1. Combine milk, egg, and salt in a small bowl thoroughly.
2. Add two teaspoons of coconut oil into a non-stick skillet and place over medium heat to melt.
3. Pour the egg mix into the skillet and cook until the bottom of the mix turns set and center a bit runny.

4. Turn the omelet to the other side and cook until it turns set or 1 minute.

5. Remove it from the heat.

6. Pour into a plate.

For Topping:

7. Top the omelet with basil, avocado, and smoked salmon.

8. Spray the remaining one teaspoon of coconut oil on top of it.

9. Serve and enjoy.

Amount per serving:

Calories: 329

Total Fat 27.4g; Saturated Fat 6.1g, Cholesterol 340mg; Sodium 219mg; Total Carbohydrate 5.3g; Dietary Fiber 3.4g; Total Sugars 1.2g; Protein 17.8g; Vitamin D 31mcg; Calcium 73mg; Iron 2mg; Potassium 481mg.

Breakfast 7

CREAM MUSHROOM BREAKFAST CASSEROLE

Time: 30 Minutes

Servings: 2

Ingredients:

5 oz. Bacon (diced)

3 oz. Mushrooms (quartered)

1/2 Cup of Heavy Whipping Cream

3 oz. Cheddar cheese (shredded)

4 Eggs (large)

1/2 Teaspoon Onion powder

Salt

Pepper

Preparation:

1. Preheat your oven to 400°F.

2. Place your skillet on high heat.

3. Pour in mushrooms, bacon, and fry until both turn golden.

4. Add salt and pepper to taste.

5. Pour the mixture into a greased baking dish.

6. Mix egg, cream, butter, onions, and cheese in a medium bowl thoroughly.

7. Add Salt and pepper to the mixture for taste.

8. Add the egg mix to the content inside the baking dish.

9. Transfer the baking dish to the oven and bake until it turns golden brown on the top and the middle is set or 24 to 30 minutes.

10. Remove from the oven, serve, and enjoy.

Amount per serving:

Calories 795

Total Fat 63.7g; Saturated Fat 28.4g; Cholesterol 491mg; Sodium 2116mg; Total Carbohydrate 5g; Dietary Fiber 0.5g; Total Sugars 1.9g; Protein 49.9g; Vitamin D 205mcg; Calcium 383mg; Iron 4mg; Potassium 724mg.

BAKED BACON AVOCADO

Time: 55 Minutes

Servings: 8

Ingredients:

4 Ripe Avocado (big sizes)

8 Eggs (large)

2 Cherry Tomatoes

4 Tablespoons Fresh Chives (chopped)

1/2 Cup Bacon bits

2 Sprigs Fresh Basil

Cheddar Cheese

Pinch of Salt

Pepper

Preparation:

1. Preheat your oven to 400°F.
2. Cut and remove the seeds from the avocado.
3. Put halves of the avocado into a baking sheet.
4. With the aid of a spoon, scoop out the avocado's flesh to create a big hole.

5. Crack on egg into each hole in the avocado and be sure the yolk is not scattered.

6. Add salt and pepper to season it.

7. Top the egg with tomatoes, basil, cheese, bacon, and chives.

8. Transfer the baking sheet into the oven and bake for 25 minutes.

9. Remove them from the oven, serve, and enjoy.

Amount per serving:

Calories 290

Total Fat 25.3g; Saturated Fat 6.2g; Cholesterol 168mg; Sodium 122mg; Total Carbohydrate 10.3g; Dietary Fiber 7.2g; Total Sugars 1.7g; Protein 8.8g; Vitamin D 16mcg; Calcium 66mg; Iron 2mg; Potassium 629mg.

Breakfast 9
Butter Ham with Wrapped Cheddar Burrito

Time: 55 Minutes

Servings: 2

Ingredients:

4 Eggs (large)

2 Tablespoon Parmesan Cheese (shredded)

1 Tablespoon Butter

4 Tablespoon Scallion (sliced)

1/2 Cup Cheddar Cheese (shredded)

6 Ham (sliced)

Salt

Preparation:

1. Combine eggs, parmesan, and salt in a medium bowl thoroughly.
2. Place a medium saucepan over medium heat.
3. Then stir in butter and allow to melt.
4. Add the egg mix into the saucepan and be sure the mixture covers fully the pan.
5. Allow the mixture to cook until it becomes set.

6. Put the cheddar cheese, ham, and scallion in the center of the egg mix.

7. Cover the saucepan and allow it is cooking until the egg turns set and cheese melted or 5 minutes.

8. Remove the saucepan from the heat, and the next is to wrap the whole content together with the content.

9. Roll it well to turn to the burrito.

10. Serve and enjoy.

Amount per serving:

Calories 712

Total Fat 45.9g; Saturated Fat 19.9g; Cholesterol 518mg; Sodium 3671mg; Total Carbohydrate 11.7g; Dietary Fiber 3.6g; Total Sugars 1.1g; Protein 60.9g; Vitamin D 38mcg; Calcium 326mg; Iron 5mg; Potassium 912mg.

Breakfast 10

MILKY VEGGIE QUICHE

Time: 15 Minutes

Servings: 2

Ingredients:

4 oz. Cremini Mushrooms (sliced)

1/2 Tablespoon Butter

4 Eggs (large)

1 Shallot (medium, minced)

4 Tablespoon Whole Milk

4 Tablespoon Parmesan (fully grated)

4 Tablespoons Sun-dried Tomatoes (chopped)

Salt

Black pepper (ground)

Preparation:

1. Preheat your oven to 375°F.

2. Place a skillet over medium heat and add butter to melt.

3. Pour in mushroom and cook for 60 seconds.

4. Pour in shallot and cook again for 40 seconds.

5. Add salt and pepper to taste.
6. Remove the skillet from the heat and place it aside.
7. Mix egg, tomatoes, milk, and parmesan in a large bowl and blend thoroughly.
8. Get your pie dish and grease with oil.
9. Pour the egg mix into the pie dish and transfer to the oven for baking.
10. Bake the mix until the eggs are set or 10 to 15 minutes.
11. Allow cooling, slice, serve, and enjoy.

Amount per serving:

Calories 372

Total Fat 24.7g; Saturated Fat 13.1g; Cholesterol 378mg; Sodium 758mg; Total Carbohydrate 8.1g; Dietary Fiber 0.6g; Total Sugars 3.8g; Protein 31.8g; Vitamin D 45mcg; Calcium 596mg; Iron 2mg; Potassium 486mg.

Breakfast 11

KETO HERBAL

Time: 55 minutes

Servings: 8

Ingredients:

2 Cups Walnuts (chopped)

1/2 Cup Sesame Seeds

2 Cups Almond (chopped)

1/2 Cup Coconut Flakes (unsweetened)

4 Tablespoons Flax Seeds

1 Teaspoon Clove (ground)

4 Tablespoon Chia Seeds

1 Tablespoon Cinnamon (ground)

1/2 Cup Coconut oil (melted)

2 Eggs White (large)

2 Teaspoons Vanilla Extract

Salt

Preparation:

1. Preheat your oven to 350°F.

2. Use cooking spray to grease your baking sheet.

Making Granola:

3. Combine walnuts, coconut flakes, almonds, chia seeds, and sesame seeds in a large bowl and mix thoroughly.

4. Pour in vanilla, cloves, cinnamon, and salt to the mix.

5. Add egg white into the granola.

6. Combine the mixture until well mixed.

7. Add coconut oil and mix again well.

8. Pour the granola mix onto the baking sheet.

9. Place the baking sheet in the oven and bake until it turns golden or for 30 to 40 minutes.

10. Stirs at an interval while baking.

11. Remove from the oven and allow cooling completely.

Amount per serving:

Calories 642

Total Fat 57.6g; Saturated Fat 17.1g; Cholesterol 56mg; Sodium 43mg; Total Carbohydrate 18.3g; Dietary Fiber 13.3g; Total Sugars 1.9g; Protein 19.9g; Vitamin D 0mcg; Calcium 337mg; Iron 7mg; Potassium 539mg.

Breakfast 12

SEASONED BRUSSELS HASH

Time: 75 Minutes

Servings: 8

Ingredients:

12 Slices Bacon

1 Onion

4 Cloves Garlic (minced)

2 Teaspoon Black pepper (freshly ground)

2 lb. Brussels sprouts (Cut into 8)

1/2 Teaspoon Red Pepper flakes (crumbled)

Kosher Salt

Preparation:

1. Place skillet over medium heat, and pour in bacon.

2. Stir-fry the bacon until it turns crispy.

3. Remove the skillet from the heat and put the bacon on a paper towel plate.

4. Reserve the fat from the bacon in the skillet.

5. Place the skillet back on the heat, pour in Brussels, and onion.

6. Cook until the veggies are softened and turn to golden.
7. Add pepper, salt, and red pepper flakes to taste.
8. Pour four tablespoons of water into the veggies and cover the skillet.
9. Cook the mix until the Brussels soft, and the water has gone or 10 minutes.
10. Then pour in garlic, and stir-fry for some seconds.
11. Make eight holes in the hash with a wooden spatula's aid to see the bottom of the skillet.
12. Crack an egg into each hole and add salt and pepper to taste.
13. Cover the skillet and cook until you are satisfied.
14. Spray the bacon to the mixture in the skillet.
15. Serve and enjoy

Amount per serving:

Calories 213

Total Fat 12.4g; Saturated Fat 4.1g; Cholesterol 31mg; Sodium 707mg; Total Carbohydrate 12.9g; Dietary Fiber 4.7g; Total Sugars 3.1g; Protein 14.8g; Vitamin D 0mcg; Calcium 50mg; Iron 2mg; Potassium 637mg.

AVOCADO WITH BREAKFAST SAUSAGE

Time: 55 Minutes

Servings: 6

Ingredients:

6 Breakfast Sausage Patties

6 Eggs (large)

2 Avocado (ripe, mashed)

Chives (cut)

2 Teaspoon black pepper (freshly ground)

Hot Sauce

Salt

Preparation:

1. Prepare the breakfast sausage, as illustrated on the box.

2. Pour the avocado and breakfast sausage into a medium bowl.

3. Use the spatula to mash both the avocado and breakfast sausage in the bowl; then add salt and pepper.

4. Spray a medium skillet with cooking spray and place over medium heat.

5. Get a mason jar and spray with cooking spray.

6. Put the Mason jar at the center of the skillet.

7. Inside the Mason jar, crack an egg in it, add salt and pepper to taste.

8. Allow the egg cooking until the egg whites are firm or 3 minutes.

9. Remove the Mason jar carefully and continue cooking until you are satisfied.

10. Remove the skillet from the heat, and then add the cooked egg to the mashed avocado mix.

11. Top it with chives and hot sauce if you desire.

12. Serve and enjoy.

Amount per serving:

Calories 272

Total Fat 20.5g; Saturated Fat 5.1g; Cholesterol 189mg; Sodium 615mg; Total Carbohydrate 9.6g; Dietary Fiber 4.7g; Total Sugars 1.7g; Protein 14.9g; Vitamin D 15mcg; Calcium 55mg; Iron 2mg; Potassium 396mg.

Breakfast 14

FROZEN VEGGIE ACAI

Time: 30 Minutes

Servings: 4

Ingredients:

For Acai Mix:

2 Bananas (large)

2 Cups Pineapple chunks (frozen)

14 oz. Acai pulp (unsweetened, frozen)

1 Cup mango (froze, diced)

1/2 Cup Cold Water

2 Tablespoons Lime juice

For Topping:

Handful of Pepitas

A handful of Coconut flakes

Handful of Blueberries

8 Medium-sized Strawberries

1 Cup Mango (diced, thawed)

Bee Pollen

Preparation:

Note: Prepare the topping first before you make the acai bowl.

1. Pour the coconut flakes into a small skillet and place over medium heat.
2. Stir occasionally until it turns golden brown.
3. Remove the skillet from the heat and place it aside.
4. Pour pineapple, banana, and mango into a food processor and process until the mixture is well processed and chunky in nature.
5. Then pour the mixture into a bowl and place aside.
6. To break the acai pulp, pour it into warm water and leave until soft.
7. Then remove the shell, and there are your pulps.
8. Pour the acai into the food processor, add lime juice and 1/2 cup of cold water, and then process until consistent.
9. If desires, add more water when processing.
10. But be sure that the acai texture is thickened.
11. Transfer the acai mix into the freezer to keep it from melting if not eating immediately.
12. Pour the acai mixture into the frozen bowl.

13. Pour into frozen bowl with any of the toppings such as pepitas, coconut, or blueberries.

14. Serve and enjoy.

Amount per serving:

Calories 723

Total Fat 39.4g; Saturated Fat 32.8g; Cholesterol 6mg; Sodium 148mg; Total Carbohydrate 93.5g; Dietary Fiber 15.6g; Total Sugars 56.4g; Protein 8.5g; Vitamin D 1mcg; Calcium 188mg; Iron 15mg; Potassium 846mg.

LUNCH RECIPES

Lunch 1

ROASTED SHRIMP WITH CAULIFLOWER

Time: 30 Minutes

Servings: 3

Ingredients:

1/2 Head Cauliflower (fresh)

1/2 Tablespoons Olive oil

0.2Kg Raw Shrimps

1 1/2 tablespoons Dill (fresh, chopped)

1 Cucumber (medium size)

1/2 Cup lemon juice (fresh)

1/2 Cup Olive oil

1 Tablespoon Lemon zest (grated)

Pinch of Pepper

Pinch of Salt

Preparation:

1. Remove tails, scales, peel, and clean the shrimps.
2. Put the shrimps on a cooking sheet and spray 1/2 tablespoon of olive oil.
3. Add salt and pepper to taste.
4. Preheat your oven to 350°F.
5. Transfer the shrimps and roast until it turns opaque or 5 to 7 minutes.

Note: Don't overcook the shrimps to avoid becoming rubbery.

6. Remove the shrimps from the oven and place aside.
7. Put the cauliflower on the cutting board and cut the florets off.
8. Chop the cauliflower into smaller cuts.
9. Put the cauliflower into the microwave until it is soft or 3 minutes.
10. Remove the seeds of the cucumber and cut it into halves.
11. Put the Shrimp on the cutting board and slice into your preferred shape.
12. Mix Shrimp, cucumber, and cauliflower in a medium bowl.

13. Then stir in lemon zest and dill and mix well.

14. Add lemon juice and olive oil, and then toss to coat.

15. Add pepper and salt to taste.

16. Serve and enjoy.

Amount per serving:

Calories 143

Total Fat 4.3g; Saturated Fat 1.1g; Cholesterol 140mg; Sodium 240mg; Total Carbohydrate 9.1g; Dietary Fiber 2.1g; Total Sugars 3.7g; Protein 17.4g; Vitamin D 0mcg; Calcium 118mg; Iron 1mg; Potassium 502mg.

Lunch 2

EXOTIC CHICKEN CURRY

Time: 25 Minutes

Servings: 3

Ingredients:

1 Pound Chicken breasts (skinless, boneless, chopped)

1 Tablespoon Virgin Olive oil (extra)

2 Cloves Garlic (small, diced)

1 Yellow Onion (small, chopped)

1/2 Tablespoon Ginger (minced)

3/4 Teaspoon Paprika

1/2 Teaspoon Cumin (ground)

3/4 Teaspoon Turmeric (ground)

1/2 Teaspoon Black pepper (ground)

3/4 Teaspoon Coriander (ground)

7 oz. Tomatoes (crushed)

3/2 Cup Chicken broth (low-sodium)

1/4 Cup Heavy Cream

1/2 Tablespoon Cilantro

Salt

Basmati Rice

Preparation:

1. Pour your Basmati rice into a medium pot and place over medium heat.

2. Then add oil.

3. Pour in onion, and cook until it turns soft or 3 minutes.

4. Put the chicken in another medium pot and place it on heat and cook until the chicken's color turns pink.

6. Add garlic and ginger to the chicken and stir-fry until it brings out a good fragrance.

7. Add the remaining ingredients to the chicken and cook for some minutes.

8. Pour in tomatoes and broth and then bring to a simmer.

9. Add heavy cream to the mixture and season it with salt and pepper.

10. Pour the rice into a serving plate.

11. Top the rice with your chicken curry and garnish with cilantro.

12 Serve and enjoy.

Amount per serving:

Calories 646

Total Fat 21.1g; Saturated Fat 6.4g; Cholesterol 148mg; Sodium 580mg; Total Carbohydrate 58.7g; Dietary Fiber 3.2g; Total Sugars 4g; Protein 52.4g; Vitamin D 5mcg; Calcium 84mg; Iron 4mg; Potassium 860mg.

Lunch 3

LIME AVOCADO SALAD

Time: 20 minutes

Servings: 4

Ingredients:

2 Ripe Avocado (small)

2 Tablespoons Lime Juice

1/2 Teaspoon Sea salt

3 Tablespoons Cilantro (fresh)

6 Eggs (large, hard-boiled, diced)

2 Tablespoons Celery (chopped)

2 Tablespoons Red onion (minced)

3/4 Tablespoon Jalapenos (minced)

Preparation:

1. Mash the ripe avocado in a medium bowl.

2. Then stir in lime juice, sea salt, and mix well.

3. Pour in red onion, cilantro, celery, and jalapenos to the mixture and mix thoroughly.

4. Then add the hard-boiled eggs.

5. Serve and enjoy.

Amount per serving:

Calories 308

Total Fat 26.2g; Saturated Fat 6.2g; Cholesterol 246mg; Sodium 336mg; Total Carbohydrate 11.7g; Dietary Fiber 7.1g; Total Sugars 1.7g; Protein 10.4g; Vitamin D 23mcg; Calcium 53mg; Iron 2mg; Potassium 625mg.

Lunch 4

GARNISHED GROUND BEEF & ZUCCHINI

Time: 15 minutes

Servings: 4

Ingredients:

0.73kg Ground beef

3/4 Teaspoon Sea salt

Pinch of Black pepper

2 Zucchini (small-sized)

2 Cloves Garlic (medium, diced)

1/2 Cup Basil pesto

1 1/2 Tablespoons Fresh Parsley (chopped)

11/2 Cup Goat cheese (crumbled)

Pinch of Black pepper

Preparation:

1. Place your skillet over medium heat, and pour in garlic.

2. Stir-fry the garlic until soft and add ground beef.

3. Season it with sea salt and pepper.

4. Use your spoon to break it apart occasionally until it turns brown.
5. Add zucchini and cook for 3 to 4 minutes.
6. Stir occasionally to become soft and turns golden.
7. Remove the skillet from the heat and add basil pesto.
8. Garnish it with goat cheese and fresh parsley.

Amount per serving:

Calories 534

Total Fat 25.4g; Saturated Fat 13.9g; Cholesterol 204mg; Sodium 618mg; Total Carbohydrate 4.8g; Dietary Fiber 1.2g; Total Sugars 2.6g; Protein 68.7g; Vitamin D 0mcg; Calcium 375mg; Iron 36mg; Potassium 1034mg.

Lunch 5

CURRY CHICKEN

Time: 30 Minutes

Servings: 4

Ingredients:

3 Chicken Breasts (skinless, boneless, thin-cut)

1 1/2 Teaspoons Garlic powder

2 Teaspoons Italian seasoning

2 Tablespoon Virgin Olive oil (extra)

1/2 Red onion (small, diced)

3 Ripe Tomatoes (diced)

1 Clove Garlic (minced)

1/4 Cup Fresh Basil (chopped)

Handful of Basil leaves (to garnish)

Balsamic vinegar

Parmesan cheese (grated)

Kosher salt

Pinch of Black pepper

Preparation:

1. Pour garlic powder, salt, pepper, and Italian seasoning in a medium bowl.
2. Pour 1 1/2 tablespoons of olive oil in a skillet and place over medium heat.
3. Put the chicken in the skillet and cook until it becomes brown.
4. In another small bowl, combine the remaining olive oil, tomatoes, red onion, basil, and garlic and mix thoroughly.
5. Divide the tomatoes mix among the chicken, then pour in balsamic vinegar, basil, and parmesan to garnish.
6. Serve immediately and enjoy.

Amount per serving:

Calories 348

Total Fat 19g; Saturated Fat 5.4g; Cholesterol 109mg; Sodium 269mg; Total Carbohydrate 6.7g; Dietary Fiber 1.6g; Total Sugars 3.5g; Protein 37.4g; Vitamin D 0mcg; Calcium 159mg; Iron 2mg; Potassium 526mg.

Lunch 6

BLUE CHEESE SALAD AND STEAK

Time: 10 minutes

Servings: 2

Ingredients:

4 Cups Romaine lettuce (chopped)

8 oz. Steak (sliced)

2 Tablespoons Balsamic Vinegar

2 Tablespoons Red onion

1/3 cup Blue cheese

2 Ripe Tomatoes (wedged)

Preparation:

1. Pour the lettuce into a medium mixing bowl.

2. Pour the balsamic vinegar on the lettuce and mix well.

3. On another plate lay the salad.

4. Place the red onions and tomatoes around the lettuce.

5. Put the sliced steak over the salad and top it with blue cheese.

6. Serve and enjoy.

Amount per serving:

Calories 349

Total Fat 12.6g; Saturated Fat 6.2g; Cholesterol 119mg; Sodium 378mg; Total Carbohydrate 9.7g; Dietary Fiber 2.4g; Total Sugars 4.9g; Protein 47.5g; Vitamin D 0mcg; Calcium 141mg; Iron 7mg; Potassium 909mg.

Lunch 7

SPICED BEEFLESS GROUND BEEF & RICED CAULIFLOWER

Time: 30 minutes

Servings: 2

Ingredients:

1/2 Recipe Beefless Ground Beef

6 oz. Riced Cauliflower (frozen)

1/2 Teaspoon taco seasoning (saltless)

2 Teaspoons Olive oil

1/2 Cup Avocado (diced)

1/2 Cup Red Cabbage (sliced)

2 Tablespoons Cilantro (fresh)

1/4 Cup Salsa

Preparation:

1. Prepare the Beefless Ground Beef according to the instruction on the box.

2. Prepare the riced cauliflower according to the instruction on the box.

3. Then add taco and olive oil to the riced cauliflower and stir.

4. Divide the riced cauliflower among tow serving containers with covers.

5. Divide beefless ground beef, cabbage, and avocado onto the tops of the riced cauliflower in containers.

6. Then add cilantro and salsa to garnish.

7. Cover the serving containers and transfer to the fridge till you are ready.

Amount per serving:

Calories 278

Total Fat 18.3g; Saturated Fat 5g; Cholesterol 14mg; Sodium 558mg; Total Carbohydrate 18.7g; Dietary Fiber 5.5g; Total Sugars 3.5g; Protein 12.1g; Vitamin D 0mcg; Calcium 101mg; Iron 2mg; Potassium 427mg.

Lunch 8

PALEO CHICKEN SALAD

Time: 40 minutes

Servings: 4

Ingredients:

2 Tablespoons Virgin Olive oil (extra)

2 Teaspoons Balsamic vinegar

1 Tablespoon Dijon mustard

1 Romaine lettuce (chopped)

1/2 Teaspoon salt

1/4 Teaspoon Black pepper

1 Clove of Garlic (pressed)

2 Eggs (hard-boiled, quartered)

6 Slices of Bacon (crumbled)

1 Cup Chicken breasts (cooked, diced)

2 oz. Blue Cheese (crumbled)

1 Avocado (ripe)

1 Tomato (ripe, diced)

Preparation:

1. Blend balsamic vinegar, olive oil, mustard, salt, and pepper in a large bowl thoroughly, and place aside.
2. Put the romaine lettuce on a serving plate.
3. Then distribute the following ingredients (cheese, eggs, avocado, tomato, chicken, and bacon) around and on top of the lettuce.
4. Pour the balsamic mix over the lettuce mix.
5. Serve and enjoy

Amount per serving:

Calories 490

Total Fat 38g; Saturated Fat 11g; Cholesterol 155mg; Sodium 1263mg; Total Carbohydrate 10.4g; Dietary Fiber 4.6g; Total Sugars 2.3g; Protein 28.4g; Vitamin D 8mcg; Calcium 109mg; Iron 5mg; Potassium 794mg.

Lunch 9

SPICY-SOUR CHICKEN

Time: 15 minutes

Servings: 2

Ingredients:

0.2kg Chicken breasts (skinless, boneless, cubed)

1/4 Cup green bell pepper (sliced)

1 Tablespoon Coconut oil

1/2 Cup Carrot (strips)

4 oz. Pineapple chunks (reserve juice)

1 Clove Garlic (small, minced)

2 Tablespoons Soy sauce (low sodium)

1/2 Tablespoon Vinegar

Pinch of Ginger (ground)

1/2 Tablespoon Brown sugar

1/4 Cup Red bell pepper (sliced)

1/2 Tablespoon cornstarch

Preparation:

1. Pour the coconut oil into a medium skillet and place over medium heat.

2. Add the chicken and cook until it turns brown.

3. Pour in green bell pepper, red bell pepper, garlic, carrot, and sauté until they are soft or 60 seconds.

4. Mix cornstarch and soy sauce in a small bowl well.

5. Pour the mixture into the skillet; then add vinegar, ginger, pineapple liquid, and sugar.

6. Mix to blend thoroughly.

7. Allow the mixture boiling for some minutes.

8. Remove the skillet from the heat.

9. Serve and enjoy.

Amount per serving:

Calories 323

Total Fat 14.4g; Saturated Fat 7.9g; Cholesterol 89mg; Sodium 1011mg; Total Carbohydrate 17.7g; Dietary Fiber 2g; Total Sugars 10.5g; Protein 30.9g; Vitamin D 0mcg; Calcium 42mg; Iron 2mg; Potassium 494mg.

Lunch 10

CREAMY KETO SALAD

Time: 10 minutes

Servings: 2

Ingredients:

To Prepare Salad:

1 Carrot (medium, shredded)

2 Heads Broccoli (cut into small sizes)

1/4 Red onion (sliced)

1/4 Cup Almonds (sliced)

1/4 Cup Cranberries (dried)

4 Slices of Bacon (cooked, crumbled)

Kosher salt

To prepare Dressing:

1 1/2 Tablespoons Apple cider vinegar

1/4 Cup Mayonnaise

Pinch of Black pepper (ground)

Kosher salt

Preparation:

1. Pour 2 cups of water and pinch of salt into a

medium sauce and place over medium heat.

2. Bring the water to a boil.

3. Pour ice water into a bowl and place it aside.

4. Once the water in the sauce boils, then pour in broccoli and cook until soft or 60 seconds.

5. Use the slotted spoon to remove the broccoli florets and place them inside the ice water bowl.

6. Allow the broccoli cooling. Drain it with the aid of a colander.

7. Blend broccoli, carrots, red onion, cranberries, bacon, and almonds in a large bowl thoroughly.

For the Dressing:

8. Combine vinegar, mayonnaise, salt, and pepper in a bowl well.

9. Serve and enjoy.

Amount per serving:

Calories 448

Total Fat 31.9g; Saturated Fat 7.1g; Cholesterol 49mg; Sodium 2396mg; Total Carbohydrate 21.8g; Dietary Fiber 5.4g; Total Sugars 6.6g; Protein 19.8g; Vitamin D 0mcg; Calcium 99mg; Iron 2mg; Potassium 742mg

Lunch 11

BEEF BURGER & KETO SAUCE

Time: 15 minutes

Servings: 2

Ingredients:

To prepare Dressing:

1/4 Cup Virgin Olive oil (extra)

1 1/2 Tablespoons Dijon mustard

3 Tablespoons Balsamic vinegar

1 Teaspoon Honey

1 Clove garlic (small, minced)

Kosher salt

Black pepper (freshly ground)

To prepare Burger:

0.2kg Organic Ground beef (grass-fed)

1 Ripe Tomato (sliced)

1 Ripe Avocado (sliced)

1/2 Teaspoon Worcestershire sauce

Pinch of Chili powder

Pinch of Onion powder

1/2 package Butter-head lettuce

1 Red onion (small, cut into rounds)

Kosher salt

Black pepper (ground)

Preparation:

To Prepare Dressing:

1. Combine all the dressing ingredients in a bowl thoroughly.

To Prepare Burger:

2. Mix Worcestershire sauce, beef, chili powder, and onion powder thoroughly.

3. Separate the burger into two patties.

4. Next is to place a grill pan over medium heat.

5. Allow the grill pan to get hot.

6. Then pour in onion and cook until it turns tender or some minutes.

7. Remove the tendered onion from the pan and add burgers.

8. Cook the burgers until they turn seared on all sides.

9. Pour lettuce and half of the dressing mix on top of it.

10. Get two serving plates and place burger patty, avocado, tomato slices, and grilled onion in each plate.

11. Pour the remaining dressing into the plates

12. Serve and enjoy.

Amount per serving:

Calories 662

Total Fat 51.7g; Saturated Fat 10.1g; Cholesterol 89mg; Sodium 598mg; Total Carbohydrate 19.7g; Dietary Fiber 8.8g; Total Sugars 7g; Protein 33.8g; Vitamin D 0mcg; Calcium 42mg; Iron 20mg; Potassium 1090mg.

MILKY CREAMY CAULIFLOWER

Time: 30 Minutes

Servings: 4

Ingredients:

1 Cauliflower (budded)

1 Teaspoon Black pepper (ground)

1/4 Cup Cheddar cheese (shredded)

3 Tablespoons Butter

1/4 Cup Almond milk (unsweetened)

1/2 Cup Heavy Cream

Kosher salt

Preparation:

1. Preheat your oven to 450°F.

2. Pour two tablespoons of butter on a baking sheet lined with foil.

3. Mix melted butter and cauliflower in a large bowl.

4. Add salt and pepper to taste.

5. Place the cauliflower florets on the prepared baking sheet.

6. Transfer it to the oven and allow roasting until it becomes crisp-tender or 12 to minutes.

7. Remove from the oven and set aside.

8. Pour cheddar cheese, heavy cream, milk, and the remaining butter into a skillet and place over medium heat.

9. Pour the cheese mix over the cauliflower.

Amount per serving:

Calories 228

Total Fat 20.3g; Saturated Fat 13.6g; Cholesterol 51mg; Sodium 195mg; Total Carbohydrate 9.3g; Dietary Fiber 4.1g; Total Sugars 4g; Protein 5.4g; Vitamin D 15mcg; Calcium 100mg; Iron 1mg; Potassium 502mg.

Lunch 13

SPICED CHICKEN & AVOCADO ASPARAGUS SALAD

Time: 10 Minutes

Servings: 2

Ingredients:

3/4 pound Asparagus (thin, trimmed)

1 Ripe Avocado (peeled, seeded, cubed)

1/2 pound Organic Chicken (cooked, cut into bite-sized)

1/2 Tablespoon Shallots (minced)

2 Tablespoons extra virgin Olive oil

1 1/2 Tablespoons Lemon juice

1/2 Teaspoon Dijon mustard

1/2 Tablespoon fresh Dill (chopped)

Sea salt

Black pepper

Preparation:

1. Pour 1 cup of water in a medium skillet and place over medium heat.

2. Then add a pinch of salt and allow it to get warm.

3. Place the asparagus in the bottom of the skillet and cover it.

4. Allow the asparagus to cook well or 3 minutes.

5. Remove the skillet from the heat and drain the water.

6. Remove the asparagus and cut it into pieces.

To make the dressing:

7. Mix shallots, dill, Dijon, and lemon in a bowl thoroughly.

8. Then season the combination with salt and pepper.

9. Pour in chicken in the dressing and mix well.

10. Then pour in asparagus and mix again well.

11. Top your meal with avocado.

12. Serve and enjoy.

Amount per serving:

Calories 538

Total Fat 37.4g; Saturated Fat 7.2g; Cholesterol 87mg; Sodium 333mg; Total Carbohydrate 16.4g; Dietary Fiber 10.5g; Total Sugars 4g; Protein 38.9g; Vitamin D 0mcg; Calcium 84mg; Iron 6mg; Potassium 1094mg.

Lunch 14

FINGER-LICKING CHICKEN SALAD

Time: 10 minutes

Servings: 4

Ingredients:

1 Cup Chicken (cooked, shredded)

1/4 Cup Greek Yogurt (plain)

1/4 Cup Celery (chopped)

1/4 Cup Apple (chopped)

1/4 Cup Pecan walnuts (toasted)

2 Tablespoons red onion (chopped)

Pinch of garlic powder

Pinch of salt

Pinch of black pepper

Preparation:

1. Mix yogurt, salt, garlic powder, and pepper in a bowl well.

2. Stir in chicken, red onion, apple, and celery into the mixture, and mix thoroughly.

3. Check if you are satisfied with the taste.

4. Serve with bread or on croissants, or it can be wrapped in lettuce.

Amount per serving:

Calories 122

Total Fat 3.6g; Saturated Fat 0.8g; Cholesterol 28mg; Sodium 91mg; Total Carbohydrate 10.9g; Dietary Fiber 1.1g; Total Sugars 2.1g; Protein 12.7g; Vitamin D 0mcg; Calcium 24mg; Iron 1mg; Potassium 133mg.

DINNER RECIPES

Dinner 1

SPICED CHICKEN & AVOCADO SALAD

Time: 40 Minutes

Servings: 4

Ingredients:

4 Chicken breasts (skinless, boneless)

1 Teaspoon Chili powder

1 Teaspoon Paprika

1/4 Cup Olive oil

1 Teaspoon Cumin

1 Teaspoon garlic powder

4 Cups Romaine lettuce

1 Red onion (medium, diced)

2 Ripe Tomatoes (diced)

2 Cilantro (fresh)

1 Cup Cucumber (cut into your shape)

4 Ripe Avocados (medium, sliced)

2 Tablespoons Olive oil

Salt

Pepper

Preparation:

1. First, wash the chicken and pat dry with paper towels.
2. Combine chili powder, cumin, garlic powder, salt, olive oil, one teaspoon of salt, and one teaspoon of pepper thoroughly.
3. Place the spices mix evenly on all sides of the chicken breasts.
4. Put two tablespoons of olive oil in a large skillet and place over medium heat.
5. Put the chicken breasts in the skillet, and occasionally flip them until the pink color is gone.
6. Remove the skillet from the heat.
7. Blend lettuce, onion, tomato, cucumber, and oil in a large bowl well.
8. Then add salt and pepper to season it.
9. Also, pour in cilantro and mix again with tongs.

10. Cut the chicken and put on top of the salad.
11. Put the sliced avocado on top of it.
12. Serve and enjoy

Amount per serving:

Calories 899

Total Fat 70.3g; Saturated Fat 14.1g; Cholesterol 130mg; Sodium 196mg; Total Carbohydrate 26.6g; Dietary Fiber 16.1g; Total Sugars 5.2g; Protein 47.9g; Vitamin D 0mcg; Calcium 79mg; Iron 6mg; Potassium 1726mg.

Dinner 2

BAKED MEATY ZUCCHINI WITH PESTO SAUCE

Time: 25 minutes

Servings: 6

Ingredients:

0.2Kg Zucchini

0.45kg Ground Beef

1 1/2 Tablespoons Olive oil

2 Cloves Garlic (minced)

1 Cup Basil pesto

1 1/2 Cups Mozzarella cheese (shredded)

1 Egg (medium)

1/4 Cup Parmesan cheese (grated)

6 oz. Ricotta cheese (grated)

Kosher salt

Preparation:

1. Preheat your oven to 400°F.

2. Slice the zucchini thinly.

3. Then lay the sliced zucchini in a single layer on a baking sheet.

4. Brush the zucchini with one tablespoon of olive oil on all sides.

5. Then spray salt lightly to all sides.

6. Transfer the zucchini to the oven and roast until it becomes soft and almost dry.

7. Remove from the oven and pat dry with a paper towel to get rid of excess oil.

8. Next is to pour 1/2 tablespoon of olive in a skillet and place over medium heat.

9. Pour in garlic and cook until tender or some seconds.

10. Add beef and cook until it becomes browned or 5 minutes.

11. Then stir in pesto sauce and mix well.

12. Remove from the heat.

13. Combine egg, ricotta, and parmesan cheese in a medium bowl thoroughly.

14. Finally, pour the zucchini slices into the glass casserole.

15. Divide the meat sauce and pour half on top of the zucchini.

16. Use a spoon to spread the ricotta cheese mix on top of it.

17. Next is to pour half of the shredded mozzarella on top also.

18. Do the layers again, but make sure it is the shredded mozzarella on the top.

19. Transfer the casserole to the oven and bake until it becomes golden brown and the cheese on top is melted or 10 minutes.

20. Garnish with basil.

Amount per serving:

Calories 258

Total Fat 13.3g; Saturated Fat 5.2g; Cholesterol 111mg; Sodium 232mg; Total Carbohydrate 3.4g; Dietary Fiber 0.5g; Total Sugars 0.8g; Protein 30.3g; Vitamin D 3mcg; Calcium 147mg; Iron 15mg; Potassium 456mg.

Dinner 3

SEASONED COD TACOS & CABBAGE SLAW

Time: 45 minutes

Servings: 4

Ingredients:

For Tacos:

10 Tortillas

4 Cod Fillets (medium)

1 Tablespoon garlic powder

2 Teaspoons Paprika

1/2 Teaspoon of cayenne pepper

1/2 Teaspoon Oregano (ground)

1 Teaspoon Mustard (dried)

1/2 Teaspoon Cumin

2 Teaspoons Kosher salt

1/4 Teaspoon Black pepper

For cabbage slaw:

2 Jalapeno (diced)

3 Cups Purple cabbage (shreddedo

2 Limes (juiced)

1 Tablespoon Olive oil

1/4 Cup Cilantro

1/2 Cup Radish (thinly sliced, halved)

2 Teaspoons Apple cider vinegar

1 Teaspoon Sea salt

Preparation:

1. Defrost the cod, as illustrated in the package directions.

2. Once the fish is defrosted, add all the ingredients for seasoning the fish in a bowl.

3. Add the fish to the mixture, blend well, and transfer to the fridge for another 15 minutes.

4. Spray a pan with cooking spray and place over medium heat.

5. Put the fish on the pan and cook all until it becomes opaque and flakey.

6. Remove the fish from the pan and cut into bitable sizes.

To prepare cabbage slaw:

7. Combine all the ingredients for cabbage slaw in a bowl thoroughly.

To prepare Tacos:

8. Pour the tortillas into a skillet and place over low heat.

9. Once they slightly char, remove them from the heat.

10. Place the tortillas on a serving plate.

11. Put the cabbage slaw over the tortilla and top it again with some fish pieces.

12. Next is to also top it with the remaining ingredients.

13. Then add Mexican cheese, guacamole, and sliced avocado.

14. Enjoy.

Amount per serving:

Calories 298

Total Fat 6.9g; Saturated Fat 0.8g; Cholesterol 55mg; Sodium 1861mg; Total Carbohydrate 37.8g; Dietary Fiber 7g; Total Sugars 3.7g; Protein 25.3g; Vitamin D 0mcg; Calcium 106mg; Iron 2mg; Potassium 365mg.

Dinner 4

PALEO PIE DINNER

Time: 15 minutes:

Servings: 2

Ingredients:

1/2 pound ground beef

1/2 Head Cauliflower (Cut into pieces)

2 Tablespoons Olive oil

1/2 Cup carrot (diced)

1 Cup Water

1 Clove Garlic (minced)

2 Tablespoons White onion (diced)

1 Red bell pepper (seeded, diced)

1 Cup Asparagus (cut into pieces)

1/4 Teaspoon Cumin (ground)

1/4 teaspoon Sea salt

1/4 Teaspoon Coriander

Pinch of Black pepper

Pinch of Paprika

Pinch of Red pepper flakes

Preparation:

1. Put 3/4 tablespoon of olive oil in a pot and place over medium heat.
2. Allow it to get hot, then put the cauliflower florets and cook until it becomes golden.
3. Add water and reduce the heat to low, and then cover the pot.
4. Then, continuing cooking until the cauliflower is soft.
5. Then remove from the heat, and then remove the cauliflower, but keep the water.
6. Pour the cauliflower and one tablespoon of the cooking water in a blender and blend until consistency.
7. If possible, add more to make it smooth, and set aside.
8. Next is to preheat your oven to 400°F.
9. Pour 3/4 tablespoon of olive oil into a skillet and place over medium heat.
10. Once it is hot, pour in carrot and onion and fry until they are tender.

11. Then pour in asparagus, bell pepper, and garlic.

12. Pour in 1/4 of the cauliflower water and cook until they are about to soft.

13. In another skillet, pour in 1/2 tablespoon of olive oil and place over medium heat.

14. Then pour in beef and cook until it turns brown.

15. Use a slotted spoon to transfer the beef to the skillet that contains vegetables.

16. Then add salt, cumin, coriander, red and black pepper.

17. Mix thoroughly.

18. Pour the mixture into a dish casserole, then pour mashed cauliflower on it.

19. Lastly, spray paprika on it.

20. Enjoy

Amount per serving:

Calories 399

Total Fat 21.5g; Saturated Fat 4.7g; Cholesterol 101mg; Sodium 172mg; Total Carbohydrate 15g; Dietary Fiber 4.9g; Total Sugars 7.7g; Protein 38.3g; Vitamin D 0mcg; Calcium 58mg; Iron 24mg; Potassium 1025mg.

Dinner 5

CREAMY ZUCCHINI

Time: 50 Minutes

Servings: 3

Ingredients:

1/2 Pound Ground Chicken (lean)

1 Zucchini (medium)

1/4 Onion (medium, chopped)

1/2 Tablespoon Olive oil

1/4 Teaspoon Paprika

Pinch of Oregano

Pinch of Black pepper (ground)

1/2 small onions (chopped)

1/2 Teaspoon Chili powder

1 Cup Cheddar cheese

1/4 Teaspoon Garlic powder

1/4 Cup Sour cream (low-fat)

1/4 Teaspoon Cumin

1 Small Jalapeno pepper (sliced)

1/4 Cup Pico de Gallo

2 Green Onions (chopped)

1/4 teaspoon Sea salt

Preparation:

1. Cut the zucchini with a mandolin slice to 1/4 inch.

2. Put the zucchini into a colander, pour salt on it, and mix well.

3. Allow the zucchini to drain for 20 minutes.

4. Preheat your oven to 400°F.

5. Lay the parchment paper inside the baking dish.

6. Pour oil into a skillet and place over medium heat.

7. Pour in onions and fry until tender or 2 minutes.

8. Then stir in chicken and cook for 5 minutes or until it becomes brown.

9. While cooking, break the chicken into small crumbles.

10. Get rid of the accumulated liquid.

11. Return the skillet with chicken to low heat, and pour in cumin, chili pepper, paprika, oregano, salt, and black pepper.

12. Combine thoroughly.

13. Remove the skillet from the heat.

14. Next, has put the zucchini slices in a layer inside the baking pan.
15. Place the pan in the oven and bake for 3 minutes.
16. Remove the zucchini from the oven, and top it with cheese and chicken mix.
17. Return to oven and bake until the cheddar cheese melts or 3 minutes.
18. Put sour cream, Pico de Gallo, jalapeno, and green onions on top of it.
19. Enjoy.

Amount per serving:

Calories 389

Total Fat 24.8g; Saturated Fat 12.4g; Cholesterol 115mg; Sodium 609mg; Total Carbohydrate 7.4g; Dietary Fiber 1.7g; Total Sugars 3.5g; Protein 33.3g; Vitamin D 5mcg; Calcium 329mg; Iron 2mg; Potassium 490mg.

Dinner 6

KETO TOMATO SOUP & CHICKEN

Time: 40 Minutes

Servings: 3

Ingredients:

0.2 Kg Ground Chicken

1/2 Tablespoon Olive oil

3 Cloves Garlic (medium, minced)

1/2 Tablespoon Italian seasoning

1/2 Quart Chicken broth

1/2 Teaspoon Fennel seeds

57 oz. Can Tomatoes (Crush)

1 Small Onion (diced)

1/2 Bunch of Kale (fresh, chopped)

1 Zucchini (small, sliced)

1 Tablespoon Tomato paste

1/2 Cup Heavy cream

4 Basil leaves (fresh, ribboned)

1/2 Head Cauliflower (small, florets)

Parmesan cheese

1/2 Teaspoon Kosher salt

Pinch of Red pepper flakes

Preparation:

1. Pour chicken, onions, garlic, and Italian seasoning in a large soup pot and place over medium heat.
2. Cook the mixture until the chicken becomes brown and onions turn soft.
3. Drain the excess fat from the mixture.
4. Return the mixture to the heat, and then pour in tomato paste, chicken broth, and crushed tomatoes.
5. Blend the mixture well, and allow boiling.
6. Then add salt for taste, and simmer for 10 minutes.
7. Add cauliflower, heavy cream, kale, and zucchini.
8. Cook until the cauliflower turns soft or 5 minutes.
9. Serve your meal with parmesan cheese and red pepper flakes (optional).

Amount per serving:

Calories 533

Total Fat 18.2g; Saturated Fat 7.8g; Cholesterol 95mg; Sodium 2524mg; Total Carbohydrate 52.4g; Dietary Fiber 12.1g; Total Sugars 23.4g; Protein 43.9g; Vitamin D 10mcg; Calcium 441mg; Iron 5mg; Potassium 985mg

Dinner 7

CREAMY AVOCADO WITH BACON OMELET

Time: 10 Minutes

Servings: 4

Ingredients:

1 Tablespoon Butter

4 oz. Goat cheese (crumbled)

6 Eggs (medium, whisked)

4 Strips Bacon (cooked, thick-cut)

1 Ripe Avocado (medium)

Microgreens

Sea salt

Ground pepper

Preparation:

1. Pour butter into a skillet and place over medium heat.

2. Cook until the butter melts and twirl it to coat the skillet.

3. Pour the whisked egg to cover the bottom of the skillet.

4. Pour ground pepper and a pinch of salt on the egg.

5. Cook the content until the egg is set.

6. Gently turn the eggs with a spatula's aid and remove the skillet from the heat.

7. Divide the eggs into eight portions

8. Then pour in goat cheese, avocado, bacon into four portions of the eggs.

9. Use the remaining four portions of the eggs to cover the ones with contents.

10. Serve the eggs mix with microgreens.

Amount per serving

Calories 455

Total Fat 37.3g; Saturated Fat 15.5g; Cholesterol 304mg; Sodium 770mg; Total Carbohydrate 6g; Dietary Fiber 3.5g; Total Sugars 1.4g; Protein 25.1g; Vitamin D 25mcg; Calcium 303mg; Iron 3mg; Potassium 454mg.

Dinner 8

CREAMY CHICKEN & MUSHROOM SAUCE

Time: 35 minutes

Servings: 6

Ingredients:

6 Chicken breasts (skinless, boneless, grated)

3/4 Cup Cremini Mushrooms (sliced

1 Cup Milk

3/4 Cup Onions (diced)

2 Cloves Garlic (minced)

3 Tablespoons Flour

3 Tablespoons Thyme leaves (fresh, chopped)

1/4 Cup Olive oil

1/2 Teaspoon Black pepper

1/2 Teaspoon Kosher salt

Preparation:

1. Add salt and pepper to the chicken for seasoning.

2. Pour 1 1/2 tablespoons of olive oil into a skillet and place over medium heat.

3. Put the chicken breasts in the skillet and cook until the chicken's color becomes golden or some minutes.

4. Reduce the heat to low and cover the skillet with a lid.

5. Cook the mixture for 15 minutes with the lid remains intact.

6. Remove the pan from the heat and allow it to rest for another 15 minutes. Leave the chicken in the skillet.

7. Put another skillet over medium heat and pour in 1 1/2 tablespoons of olive oil.

8. Add mushrooms and onion and then cook until the mushroom gives out water, and the water was evaporated or for 10 minutes.

9. Stir in flour and cook the mixture until fragrant or for 3 minutes.

10. Then pour in garlic and for 1 minute.

11. Add a quarter of the milk, thyme, salt, and pepper.

12. Then stir the mixture until it becomes thick.

13. Pour another quarter of the milk and turn again until it thickens.

14. Place the chicken on the serving plates and pour the sauce over it.

15. Enjoy.

Nutrition Facts per serving:

Amount per serving

Calories 137

Total Fat 10g; Saturated Fat 1.9g; Cholesterol 11mg; Sodium 222mg; Total Carbohydrate 8g; Dietary Fiber 1g; Total Sugars 2.6g; Protein 4.9g; Vitamin D 0mcg; Calcium 84mg; Iron 2mg; Potassium 87mg.

Dinner 9

CREAMY CRISPY ZUCCHINI FRIES

Servings: 6

Time: 45 minutes

Ingredients:

3 Zucchini

2 Eggs (large)

1/2 Teaspoon Garlic powder

1 Cup Parmesan cheese (grated)

1/2 Teaspoon Sea salt

1/2 Teaspoon Black pepper

Preparation:

1. Preheat your oven to 425°F.

2. Line a large baking sheet with parchment paper.

3. Cut one zucchini half lengthwise four times. It will be in 8 long pieces. Cut the pieces crosswise. It will bring out 16 pieces from each squash.

4. Do the same for the remaining zucchini.

5. Dry the zucchini with paper towels.

6. Crack the eggs in one bowl and whisk.

7. In another bowl, pour in cheese, garlic powder, and black pepper.

8. Dip each squash piece into the egg bowl and shake the excess egg off from it.

9. The same squash dipped inside egg should be dip into the cheese mix bowl and combine until well coated on all sides.

10. Lay the coated zucchini on the baking sheet.

11. Do the same procedure for the remaining squash.

12. Transfer them to the oven and bake, turning them and rotating the baking pan until they look dark golden.

13. Place them under the broiler until they become darker golden and crispy.

14. Serve and enjoy.

Nutrition Facts per serving:

Amount per serving:

Calories 198

Total Fat 12.3g; Saturated Fat 7.2g; Cholesterol 95mg; Sodium 1200mg; Total Carbohydrate 6.4g; Dietary Fiber 1.2g; Total Sugars 1.9g; Protein 19.1g; Vitamin D 5mcg; Calcium 557mg; Iron 1mg; Potassium 281mg.

Dinner 10

SPICED BEET PASTA WITH SPAGHETTI

Time: 1 hr. 20 minutes

Servings: 6

Ingredients:

For beet pasta and sauce:

3 Red beets (large, greens)

3/4 Cup Olive oil

1.5 Pounds Spaghetti (gluten-free)

3/4 Cup Silvered Almonds (raw)

3 Tablespoons Red wine vinegar

6 Cloves Garlic (peeled)

3 Tablespoons Oregano (dried)

2 Tablespoons Parsley (dried)

Pinch of Sea salt

For Mushrooms and Greens:

1 1/2 Tablespoons Coconut oil

1 1/2 Cups Spinach (sliced)

1 1/2 Teaspoons Garlic powder

3 3/4 Cups Cremini mushrooms (sliced)

1 1/2 Teaspoons Oregano (dried)

1 1/2 Teaspoons Kosher salt

1/2 Teaspoon black pepper (ground)

Pine nuts

Preparation:

To prepare beet sauce:

1. Preheat your oven to 400°F.

2. Remove the tops of the beet and slice the greens only.

3. Remove the beets and cut them into chunks.

4. Place the chunks on a sheet pan and sprinkle them with olive oil.

5. Transfer them to the oven, bake, and occasionally turn over with a spatula until they become tender.

To prepare pasta:

6. Add salt into a large pot and place over medium heat.

7. Bring the salty water to boil and then stir in pasta.

8. Cook until the pasta is firm.

9. Then remove the pot from the heat and set aside.

10. Pour silvered almonds and garlic in a food processor and process until smooth.

11. Then add vinegar, roasted beet, salt, oregano, parsley, and half olive oil into the food processor.

12. Pulse the mixture again until it is a smooth sauce and then place aside.

To prepare mushrooms and greens:

13. Pour coconut oil into a medium skillet and place over medium heat.

12. Then stir in mushrooms and cook until they soft and juicy or 7 minutes.

13. Pour in spinach and the sliced beet greens.

14. Cook for some minutes, and stir to make sure the greens are not wilted fully.

15. Add oregano, garlic, salt, and pepper to taste.

16. Stir again to mix thoroughly.

17. Cover the mixture and continue cooking over low heat for 3 minutes.

18. Remove the mixture from the heat and serve.

19. Enjoy

Amount per serving:

Calories 749

Total Fat 42.9g; Saturated Fat 8g; Cholesterol 83mg; Sodium 786mg; Total Carbohydrate 76g; Dietary Fiber 4.4g; Total Sugars 6.2g; Protein 19.5g; Vitamin D 0mcg; Calcium 124mg; Iron 6mg; Potassium 773mg.

Dinner 11

CREAMY ITALIAN TURKEY SALAD

Time: 20 Minutes

Servings: 2

Ingredients:

1/2 Pound Ground Turkey (lean)

1 Cup Tomatoes (fresh, chopped)

2 Tablespoons Italian seasoning

1/2 Cup Guacamole

1/2 Cup Cheddar cheese (low fat)

1/4 Cup Salsa

3 Cups romaine lettuce

Preparation:

1. Pour the turkey into a skillet and place over medium heat.

2. Cook the turkey until it is browned and occasionally stir or 5 minutes.

3. Remove the fat and stir in Italian seasoning, water.

4. Continue cooking for another 3 minutes.

5. Lay two serving plates and place equal amounts of lettuce, tomatoes, salsa, cheese, and guacamole.

6. Serve and enjoy

Amount per serving:

Calories 642

Total Fat 47.2g; Saturated Fat 12.1g; Cholesterol 155mg; Sodium 1795mg; Total Carbohydrate 22.6g: Dietary Fiber 9.3g: Total Sugars 5.6g; Protein 42.9g; Vitamin D 3mcg; Calcium 272mg; Iron 7mg; Potassium 767mg.

Dinner 12

SPAGHETTI SQUASH SHRIMP

Time: 35 Minutes

Servings: 1

Ingredients:

1 Pound Spaghetti squash

3/4 Tablespoon Olive oil

1 Clove Garlic

4 oz. raw Shrimp (minced, peeled, deveined)

3 oz. baby Spinach

Pinch of Kosher salt

Pinch of Red pepper (crushed)

Preparation:

1. Preheat your oven to 375°F.

2. Cut the ends of the squash off.

3. Trim the squash into rings.

4. Scoop out the seed and membranes out with a spoon.

5. Coat a baking sheet with foil and spray with cooking spray.

6. Lay the squash rings on the baking sheet.

7. Transfer to the oven and bake until they are tender or 25 minutes.

8. Remove the squash from the oven to allow cooling.

9. Use a knife to cut the squash open to get to the strands.

10. Scrap the strands from the squash.

11. Next is to add butter and oil to a skillet and place over medium heat.

12. Pour in pepper, garlic, and cook for some seconds.

13. Stir in shrimp and cook for one minute, then add spinach and toss well.

14. Pour in the squash strands.

15. Remove it from the heat.

16. Enjoy.

Amount per serving:

Calories 427

Total Fat 15.7g; Saturated Fat 2.7g; Cholesterol 239mg; Sodium 580mg; Total Carbohydrate 46.1g; Dietary Fiber 3.5g; Total Sugars 6.4g; Protein 32.6g; Vitamin D 0mcg; Calcium 307mg; Iron 5mg; Potassium 1393mg.

Dinner 13

SPICED AVOCADO

Time: 20 Minutes

Servings: 8

Ingredients:

1 Avocado (medium)

1 Onion (chopped)

1 Ripe Tomato (chopped)

1 Clove Garlic (minced)

1 Lime (juiced)

Pinch of Pepper

Pinch Salt

Preparation:

1. Wash the avocado well.

2. Cut it into two, get rid of the seed, and put it in a serving bowl.

3. Mash the avocado with a spatula.

4. Add onions, garlic, tomato, lime juice, salt, and pepper.

5. Transfer the bowl to the fridge for one hour.

6. Enjoy.

Amount per serving:

Calories 61

Total Fat 5g; Saturated Fat 1g; Cholesterol 0mg; Sodium 22mg; Total Carbohydrate 4.8g; Dietary Fiber 2.3g; Total Sugars 1.1g; Protein 0.8g; Vitamin D 0mcg; Calcium 10mg; Iron 0mg; Potassium 171mg.

Dinner 14

SPICY ROASTED CHICKEN

Time: 45 Minutes

Servings: 4

Ingredients:

2 Pounds Chicken (giblets removed)

1 Celery (removed leaves)

3/4 Tablespoon Onion powder

1/2 Cup Butter

Black pepper

Salt

Preparation:

1. Preheat your oven to 350°F.

2. Put your chicken on a roasting pan and season it with salt and pepper thoroughly.

3. Pour onion powder into the chicken.

4. Pour some butter inside the chicken activity.

5. Spray the remaining butter around the outside of the chicken.

6. Cut the celery into four pieces and put inside the chicken cavity.

7. Transfer the chicken to the chicken and bake for 50 minutes.

8. Set the temperature of the oven to 180F.

9. Remove the chicken from the oven and use the butter and drippings to polish.

10. over the chicken with aluminum foil.

11. Allow resting for 20 minutes.

12. Enjoy.

Amount per serving:

Calories 552

Total Fat 29.9g; Saturated Fat 16.5g; Cholesterol 236mg; Sodium 354mg; Total Carbohydrate 1.4g; Dietary Fiber 0.2g; Total Sugars 0.6g; Protein 66.2g; Vitamin D 16mcg; Calcium 45mg; Iron 2mg; Potassium 469mg.

SNACKS

Snack Day 1. Sunflower seeds and sliced Avocado.

Snack Day 2. Carrots dipped in Almond butter.

Snack Day 3. Sliced veggies cubed cantaloupe.

Snack Day 4. Pistachios and hummus.

Snack Day 5. Carrots dipped in Sunflower butter.

Snack Day 6. Protein shake.

Snack Day 7. Hard-boiled egg and veggies.

Snack Day 8. Salmon wrapped with lettuce.

Snack Day 9. Hard-boiled egg Sliced Avocado.

Snack Day 10. Sliced apple with Sunflower butter.

Snack Day 11. Hummus and a piece of fruit.

Snack Day 12. Protein bar.

Snack Day 13. Carrots dipped in Sunflower butter.

Snack Day 14. Sour Cream with sliced almonds.

Chapter 7

ENDOMORPH EXERCISES

There is no doubt that exercise is one of the critical parts of any weight loss plan. This does not exclude people with endomorph body type. Naturally, exercises aid in increasing the metabolic rate and reduction of fat.

Cardiovascular exercises, like jumping jacks, will burn calories and help in creating a calorie deficit. If you are advised to go for cardiovascular exercises, it's an indication that you are storing up more calories than is necessary, and they have to get rid of the excess fat stored.

TYPES OF TRAINING

High-intensity interval training (HIIT)

HIIT training is a kind of training that involves the ability to alternate between different kinds of phases from a very high-intensity exercise and low-intensity exercise and rest. This type of training can be done two to three times per week for people with endomorph body type, and it must not be less than 30 minutes per workout.

Steady-state training (SST)

The training pieces involved in this type of training are longer consistent and moderate to low-intensity exercise, which must be consistent if effective. The exercises in this training include swimming, jogging, and walking. For people with endomorph body type, you can use this kind by doing a 30 to 60-minute session of two to three per week.

ENDOMORPH WORKOUT

Benefits of Cardiovascular exercises for people with endomorph body type are;
• Ability to balance weight.

• Getting rid of fat around the waist.

The followings are some good cardiovascular exercise that people with endomorph body type can do at home:

Jump Rope

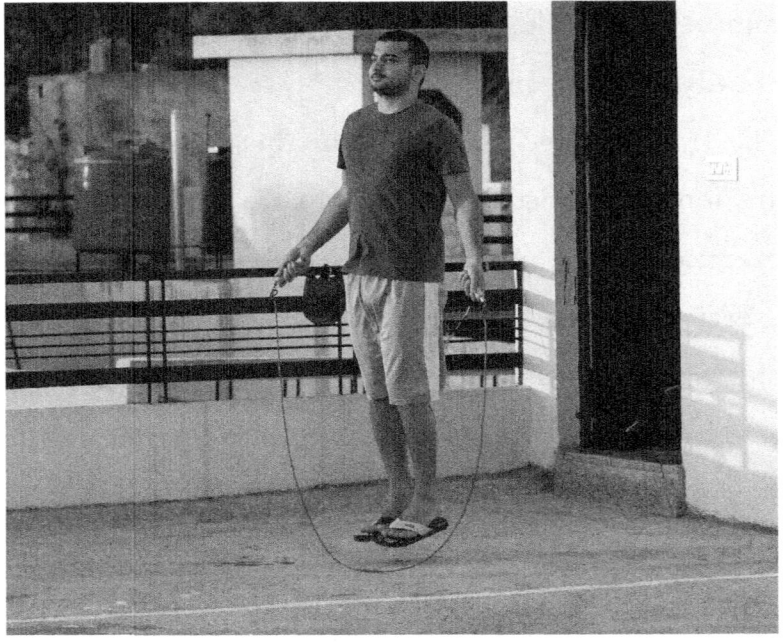

Jump rope is an excellent exercise, as it helps in burning calories. This workout is useful because it will help burn 200 to 300 calories in 13 minutes.

Benefits:

The jump rope will help in burning calories.

They help in the improvement of coordination.

Help in the reduction of injury risk.

Aids the condition of heart health.

The right way to strengthening bone density.

Steps:

1. Get a jump rope and a good pair of shoes.

2. Turn a rope with handles repeatedly while you jump over it.

3. To avoid accidents as a beginner, turn the rope with your wrists, not with your arms, and land softly.

4. Don't jump too high to avoid an accident.

5. Do continues jumping of 10 to 30 seconds for a set.

6. Do 5 sets of 10 repetitions?

Jumping Jacks

Jumping jacks are great workout tools for the total body that can be done almost anywhere. They work majorly on muscle, lungs, and heart. Jumping jacks are known to burn more than 100 calories in 10 minutes. Other parts that they affect are;

Quadriceps.

Glutes.

Hip flexors.

Shoulder muscles.

Abdominals.

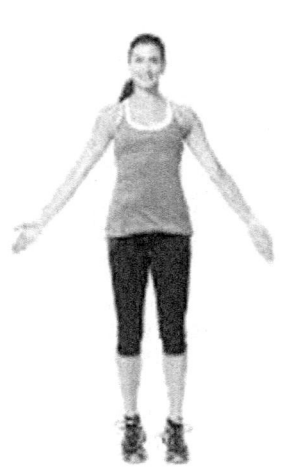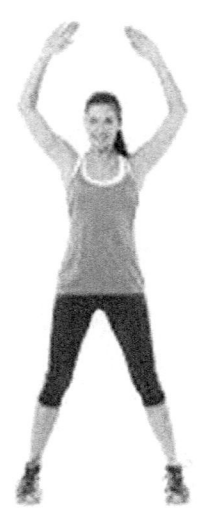

Benefits:

They help in the management of weight.

Help to reduce blood pressure.

Help to reduce and cholesterol.

Help to increase insulin sensitivity in the body.

Help to increase good cholesterol.

Steps:

1. Get a good pair of shoes.

2. Jump repeatedly while the feet apart and cycling the arms overhead.

3. Repeat for the next 45 to 60 seconds and stop.

4. Repeat until you can go for 2 minutes at a stretch.

Burpees

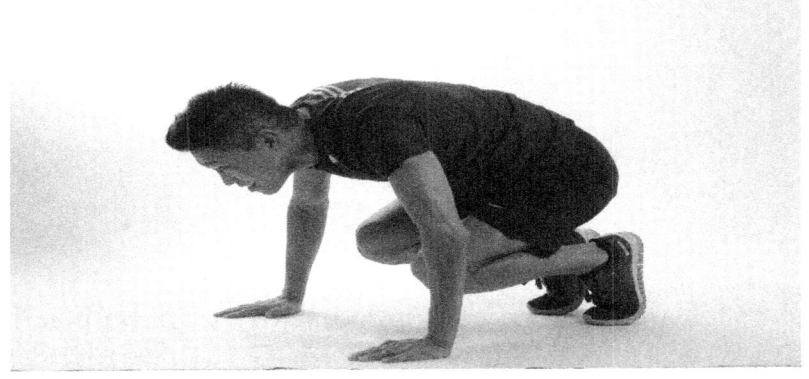

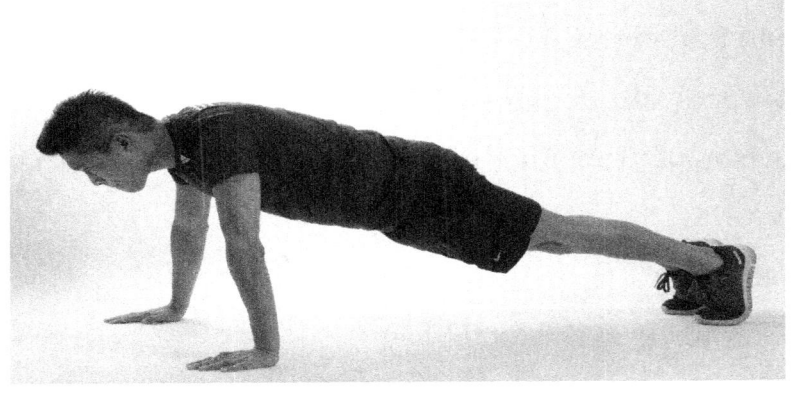

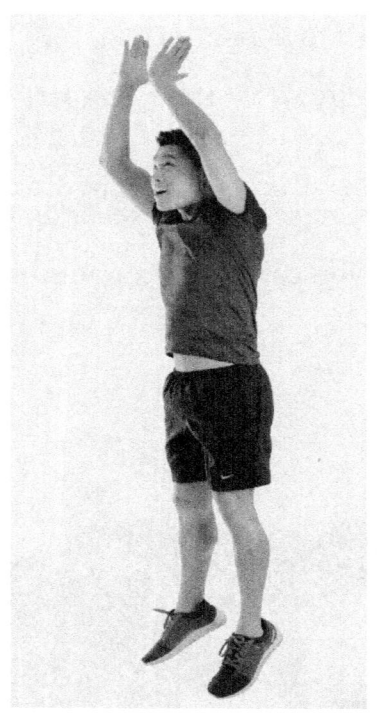

Burpees are kinds of workouts that will work on major muscle groups in the body. They are in two-part, push, and leap in the air.

Burpees are so great in burning calories that if a person of 185 pounds can do 20 minutes, it will burn 15 calories.

Benefits:

They work on the total body.

They improve cardio fitness and help in burning fats.

Burpees are versatile and convenient.

Burpees require no special equipment.

Steps:

1. Squat with knees bent, back straight, and feet about shoulder-width apart.
2. Low the hands to the floor in fronts or to inside the feet.
3. With the weight on the hands, kick feet back to be on hands and toes and in a push-up state.
4. Keep the body straight from head to heels with one push-up.
5. Don't allow the back to sag or to stick butt in the air.
6. Frog kick by jumping the feet to their former position.
7. Sit and reach the arms over the head.
8. Quickly jump into the air, so to land at the former position.
9. Once landed with the knees bent, get into the squat position, and repeat the steps.

10 Do 45 to 60 seconds of Burpees and rest for 45 to 60 seconds.

11. Repeat for 10 minutes or more.

Mountain Climbers

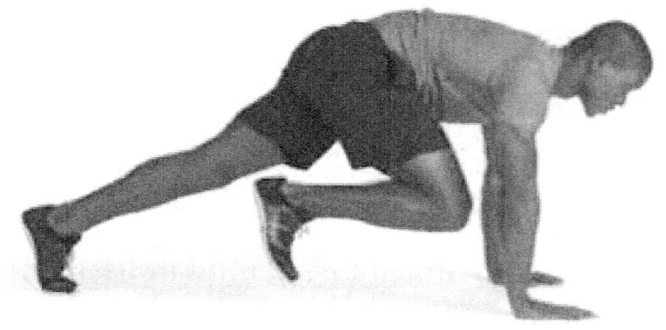

Mountain Climbing is a workout that will stretch your core and work on muscular endurance with cardio.

Mountain climbers work on wrists, shoulders, and arms.

Benefits

Improve flexibility.

Great for the butt.

Lower body strength boosters.

It can be done anywhere.

Great for the heart.

Enhanced mobility.

Great for your balance.

Burn fat.

Make you stronger.

Excellent for strengthening the core.

Steps:

1. Get down with both your arms and legs on the floor as a push-up.

2. Keep running the knees in and out from a push position.

3. Alternate left leg and right leg forward and backward.

4. Do the processes between 45 to 60 seconds.

5. Repeat the cycle in 10 minutes.

Bear Crawl Push-Ups

Bear Crawl Push-Ups is a variation of bear crawl hold that comes with push-ups. Its major work is to add extra coordination, strengthens shoulders, and help a range of muscle groups, core, and legs.

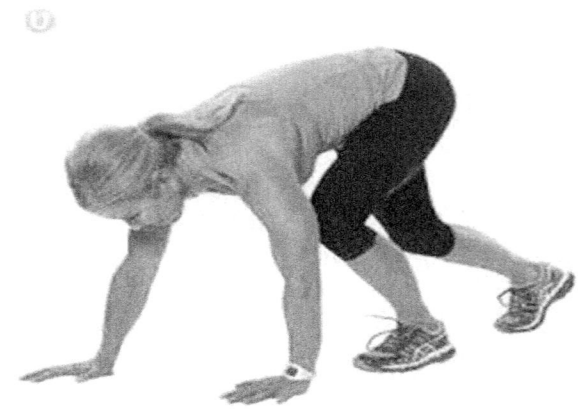

Benefits

Encourages Engagement.

Better Workout Efficiency.

Improves Athletic and Daily Performance.

May Boost Cognitive Functioning.

Steps:

1. Move forward by moving right hand and left leg forward in a crawling manner.

2. Place a weight on the right hand and left leg.

3. Then switch sides and move the left hand and right leg forward.

4. Keep your body low and continue with crawling movement.

5. Do this in 5 to 8 steps, and take a short break of 30 to 60 seconds.

Jog in Place

Jog in a place is a kind of workout that you can do anywhere, and you need little space to do it. Jog in Place is jogging while standing at a spot or in a static position.

It is a high impact exercise that will affect your joints and maybe boring at times.

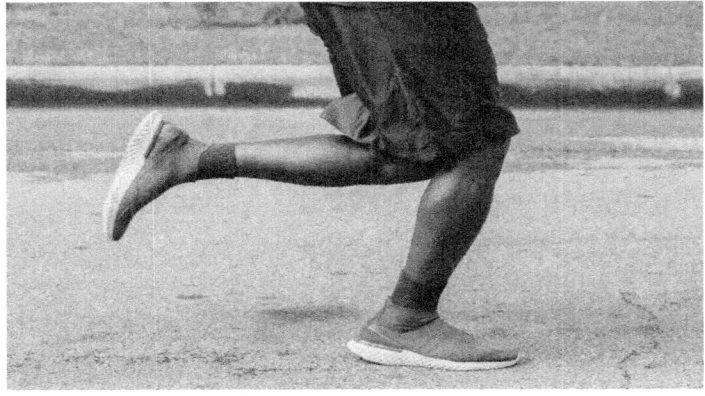

Steps:

1. Stand with your feet hip at a distance apart.

2. Raise one foot and then the other foot to jog in a place working the legs and increasing the heart rate.

Squats jumps

These are power-packed HIIT workouts. It majorly works on;

Glutes.

Lower abs.

Leg muscles.

Benefits of Squats Jump

Helps in burning calories and fat.

Ability to help in maintaining mobility and balance.

Helps in boosting sports performance.

Improvement of Health.

Improvement of bone health.

Ability to help with the removal of waste.

Helps to tone Abs muscles, legs, and butt.

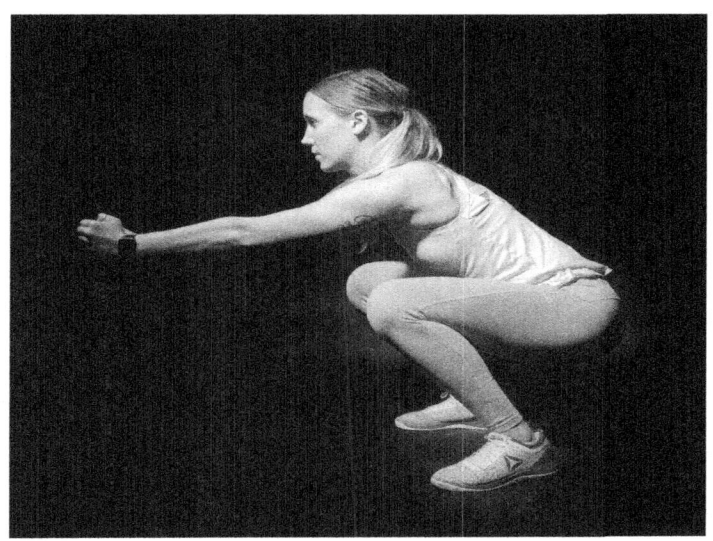

Steps:

1. Be straight on the feet apart, your hands by sides, chest up, your shoulders rolled back, chin up, and looking ahead.

2. Push the back out, bend the knees, and squat down. The knees should be above the toes. Bend forward to avoid the lower back from getting hurt and curving.

3. Bring the two hands to clap as you bend to squat down.

4. As you are about to get up, move the body upward, and jump. Then throw the hands downwards to create a big force.

5. Land gently on the land and squat.

6. S Repeat these 3 sets of 15 repetitions each.

Kickboxing

Kickboxing is a combination of kicking and punching against an object that may include a person, bag, or an air. This is a high-intensity exercise that can burn enough calories in a couple of minutes.

Benefits of Kickboxing

It helps to reduce stress.

It boosts your confidence levels.

It will aid coordination.

Kickboxing burns mega calories.

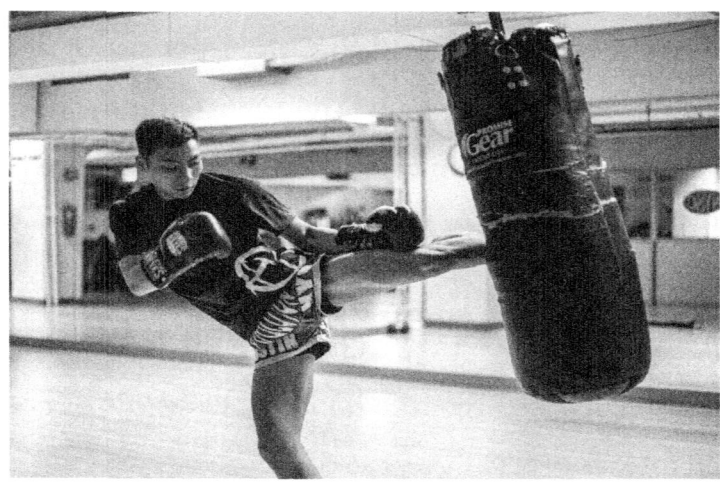

7 DAYS SAMPLE OF ENDOMORPH WORKOUT PLAN

Guidelines:

1. You are expected to do 3 to 5 sets of activities of any of the exercises listed below.

2. Pick the weight that will make you fail between 8 to 12 reps.

3. To achieve the best hormonal response, select 2 minutes slow, I minute for a fast interval workout.

High-frequency workouts

Day 1

Targeted area: Triceps/Chest

Note: It is expected to select any 3 to 5 of the activities below:

Activities:

- Pushups.
- Dumbbell Fly's.
- Weight Bench Dips.
- .Flat Barbell Bench Press.

•.Bench Press.

Day 2
Targeted area: Biceps/back
Note: It is expected to select any 3 to 5 of the activities below:

Activities:
- Seated Rows.
- .Dumbbell Hammer Curls.
- .Pull-Ups.
- .Bar Biceps Curls.
- .Bent-Over Row.
- .Deadlift.

Day 3
Targeted area: Cardio
Note: It is expected to select any 1 to 2 of the activities below:

Activities:
- Cycling.
- Step Mill.

- Swimming.

Day 4
Targeted area: Shoulders/Calves/Abs

Note: It is expected to select any 3 to 5 of the activities below:

Activities:
- Dumbbell Lateral.
- Dumbbell Rear Lateral.
- Leg Raises.
- Russian Twists.
- Dumbbell Overhead Press.
- Standing Shoulder.
- Planks.
- Cable Crunch.

Day 5
Targeted area: Quads/Hams/Glutes

Note: It is expected to select any 3 to 5 of the activities below:

Activities:

- Glute Bridges.
- Single-Leg Presses.
- Leg Extensions.
- Squats jumps.
- Dumbbell Reverse Lunges.

Day 6:

Targeted area: Cardio

Note: It is expected to select any 1 to 3 of the activities below:

Activities:
- Cycling.
- Swimming.
- Step Mill.
- Russian Twists.

Day 7:

No Workout and take rest

Chapter 8

MAINTAINING THE REQUIRED WEIGHT

The irony about losing weight is that most people who lost significant amounts of weight regain it quickly. A credible report online says that more than 80% of dieters who started a weight loss plan were not successful in their long-term goals.

However, this statistic should not deter or discourage you from pursuing your goal. The diet, workouts, and lifestyle, coupled with all the factors below, will make your goal achievable when followed religiously.

Don't Skip Breakfast.

If you have an endomorph body type, breakfast is a must for you as it will help you manage your weight. Some reports and studies support the notion that those who eat breakfast are healthier as most of them live a good lifestyle, such as exercising and eating more fiber and micronutrients. So it is recommended that the people with endomorph body type not skip breakfast, as it will not lead to weight loss.

Consume more protein

Naturally, it will take more calories to digest proteins in the food than it will take to digest other macros such as carbohydrates and fat. Proteins need more amounts of energy to be digested. The energy needed is known to be up to 30% of the calories. This statement's meaning is that you will burn up to 30% of the calories in the protein eaten for you to digest it. This process will help you reduce the number of calories your body will absorb in helping you lose weight. Proteins are promoters of muscle growth, thereby helping you burn more calories and manage weight.

Eat More Greens

To the endomorphs, it is recommended to always go for foods that will provide all the necessary nutrients with fewer calorie counts. Foods that are of low-calorie counts are vegetables, as they will help you in the management of weight and give you better health options.

Always be hydrated

Water is essential to life.

If you are starting to lose weight, is it necessary and helpful to drink enough water for weight maintenance? Water is known to aids fullness and indirectly keep the amount of calorie intake in check if you drink enough before meals. A report says that those who drank water before their meal had up to a 13% reduction in calorie consumption than those who didn't take water before a meal. Also, another credible report says that if you are the type who drinks water every time, there is a likelihood that there will be an increase in the number of calories that will be burnt throughout the day.

Monitor your Weight Regularly

It is essential to monitor your weight by climbing on a scale every on a regular basis. This scale is a tool needed for weight management, as it will let you be aware of the progress making and the encouragement to go more. If you weigh yourself every tie, you will know if you are to eat lower calories or large calorie.

Stick to Your Diet Plan

There is a common habit when it comes to diet plan, and is religiously following the plan during weekdays but cheating the plan during the weekend days. This habit is known to lead people to binge on junks that will ruin their weight management efforts. If you always found yourself in this situation and you did not try to stop, be assured that you will regain more weight than you lost during the weekdays. However, a report says that those who follow their diet during the weekend days as they do during the weekdays have greater chances of losing and maintaining their weights in the long term.

Sleep Well

Do you know that having enough sleep will affect the control of your weight? To be sincere with you, denying yourself sleep over a long period will affect your weight management. The main reason is that inadequate sleep will lead to higher hormone levels in the body, known as ghrelin. Ghrelin hormone is a hunger hormone in the body that increases appetite. If the type that doesn't sleep well, it is recommended that you adjust your sleep habits.

Join a Support Group

Maintaining a long-term goal can be difficult if done alone. One of the best ways to solve these challenges is to join a support group where everyone will be accountable. With this support group, each member will hold each other and possibly partner in the same healthy lifestyle.

Be Consistent

No doubt that to achieve a long term goal, consistency

is the key.

So if you are on the journey to control weight, consistency should be taken to the background. It is better not to have this on and off dieting habits that will lead to going to old habits. So it is advised to maintain the new habits you have to engage in to achieve your health goals.

CONCLUSION

Thank you for buying this book!

I hope you enjoy the recipes, workouts, and lifestyle recommended in this book to bring you closer to your dream. If you religiously follow the plans and recipes written in this book, you will always stay in top shape inside out.

Though it may be difficult in the beginning to adjust to eating natural foods, within some days, your taste buds will start to appreciate it once you are always on the healthy veggies. So the golden advice is to stay fit and, most importantly, stay consistent.

So, start using this book for the expected dramatic transformation of your body from endomorph to mesomorph.

Thanks

References

Tiffany Nicholas: Carb Cycling for Beginners: Simple Recipes and Exercises for Weight Loss, Reactivating Metabolism and Muscle Building

https://www.everydayhealth.com/diet-nutrition/endomorph-diet/

https://best5supplements.com/fat-burners/best-fat-burners-endomorphs/

https://www.medicalnewstoday.com/articles/325577#endomorph-exercises

https://www.healthline.com/nutrition/maintain-weight-loss

https://www.cnet.com/health/how-to-track-your-macros-guide/

https://biostrap.com/blog/what-is-the-best-macro-ratio-for-you-based-on-your-phenotype-body-shape/

Printed in Great Britain
by Amazon